ADVANCED PRACTICE NURSING

Setting a New Paradigm for Care in the 21st Century

SYDNEY LENTZ PHD

authorHOUSE®

AuthorHouse™
1663 Liberty Drive
Bloomington, IN 47403
www.authorhouse.com
Phone: 1-800-839-8640

Published by AuthorHouse 12/18/2013

ISBN: 978-1-4918-0084-3 (sc)
ISBN: 978-1-4918-0031-7 (hc)
ISBN: 978-1-4918-0030-0 (e)

Library of Congress Control Number: 2013913129

FOREWORD

As the healthcare needs of society continue to evolve, it is becoming increasingly evident that advanced practice nurses have an essential and expanding role in the provision of healthcare in the 21st century. The Patient Protection and Affordable Care Act (PPACA) of 2010, the Institute of Medicine's 2010 report, *The Future of Nursing: Leading Change, Advancing Health* (IOM 2010), and the American Nurses Association's *Nursing's Social Policy Statement* (ANA 2010) provide evidence that as society's needs evolve, nursing has both the ability and the responsibility to meet those needs.

The PPACA will ensure that more than 32 million Americans have access to healthcare. This staggering number presents a challenge for all healthcare professionals. Nursing's role involves the provision of healthcare as well as educating and counseling patients regarding preventive strategies to maintain optimal health.

In addition, the 2010 IOM report highlights the role nurses have in transforming healthcare. Specifically, this report recommends that:

- Nurses should practice to the full extent of their education and training.

- Nurses should achieve higher levels of education and training through an improved education system that promotes seamless academic progression.

- Nurses should be full partners, with physicians and other healthcare professionals, in redesigning healthcare in the United States.

- Effective workforce planning and policy making require

better data collection and an improved information infrastructure (IOM, 2010).

Finally, *Nursing's Social Policy Statement* defines the social concerns in healthcare and nursing and states that nursing has an "active and enduring leadership role in public and political determinations about the following six key areas of health care:

- The organization, delivery, and financing of quality health care;

- The provision for the public's health;

- The expansion of nursing and healthcare knowledge and appropriate application of technology; expansion of resources and health policy;

- Definitive planning for health policy and regulation; and duties under extreme conditions" (ANA, 2010, pp. 4-5).

Given the IOM's recommendations and nursing's commitment to society, advanced practice registered nurses (APRNs) are most assuredly at the forefront of healthcare in the 21st century. This very timely book thoughtfully describes the various ways in which APRNs are meeting the needs of society and healthcare.

The author offers evidence of the innovative strategies APRNs are using to provide healthcare in various settings such as delivering healthcare in rural communities, providing hospice and palliative care, increasing access to care through retail clinics, offering healthcare in schools, in the acute care setting, in a midwife hospital, and as a certified registered anesthetist. Most chapters include a reflective interview that elucidates how advanced practice nurse leaders are fulfilling the recommendations of the IOM as well as those in *Nursing's Social Policy Statement*.

It is apparent that as more Americans gain access to healthcare, more innovative strategies to provide care will be developed—and I am confident that nursing will be at the forefront of these strategies. The ANA describes most accurately how nursing will meet society's needs in the 21st century: "Nursing is the pivotal health care profession, highly valued for its specialized knowledge, skill, and caring in improving the health status of the public and ensuring safe, effective, quality care" (ANA, 2010, p. 1).

Lisa Astalos Chism, DNP, APRN, BC, NCMP, FAANP
Nurse Practitioner/Certified Menopause Practitioner
Clinical Director, Women's Wellness Clinic, Karmanos Cancer Institute

References

American Nurses Association (ANA). 2010. *Nursing's Social Policy Statement: The Essence of the Profession.* Silver Spring, MD. Available at Nursebooks.org

Institute of Medicine (IOM). (2010, October). *The Future of Nursing: Leading Change, Advancing Health.* Washington, DC. Available at www.iom.edu/Reports

PREFACE

We are facing a healthcare crisis: millions of people need both primary care and hospital care. Healthcare expenses continue to rise, and the number of primary care physicians is in sharp decline. In the face of this crisis, nurse practitioners (NPs) and other advanced practice nurses (APNs) are providing excellent patient services.

In each of these case studies, I worked to provide all NPs with their unique story, written from their viewpoint. I spent considerable time with each of the APNs profiled in this book, getting to know them and learning about their clinical practice, their specialty, and how they are working collaboratively with physicians, nurses, and other health professionals. Most important, I learned to appreciate the unique gifts that they bring to their patients, their colleagues, and their profession. Reading stories about what others have done to build a healthcare practice will help nurses realize that they too have what it takes to transform their own practices—whether they work in clinics, hospitals, universities, or public health settings. This practical guide makes it easy for nurses to glean usable ideas and apply them immediately.

My original visit with Dr. Joan Slager took place in July 2010. Joan serves as a nurse midwife at Bronson Women's Service in Kalamazoo, Michigan. I spent a day with her, learning how Bronson unwaveringly supports midwives in providing care that is less medical and more natural. Joan explained the midwifery vision, as well as the rules and regulations of The Joint Commission. She noted that midwives do not limit their activities to birthing care, but provide various kinds of wellness care for women of all ages. I learned the importance of staff- and patient-supportive scheduling and strategies for collaborating with physicians. I also was made aware of Bronson's values, which mandate treating women from all cultures with respect. I cannot presume to know all that it takes to make women understand the changes that their bodies go through as they come of age and head into their senior years.

I followed up with a visit to Jonnie Hamilton in December 2011. Jonnie serves as Director, Napoleon Jordan Center for HealthCare at Marcus Garvey Academy on Van Dyke in Detroit, Michigan. From Jonnie, I learned about school-based health care and the regulations that apply to these activities. I also learned about the importance of vaccinations, both to students and their families. I learned that Jonnie needed support from other school-based NPs and from the medical director for community health at St. John's Providence Health System to establish her school-based clinic. What I learned about myself is that I underestimated all the efforts that are necessary to provide school-aged children with what they need: good food, exercise, alternative diabetes medications, removal of asthma triggers from their homes, peak flow measurements, and strategies for navigating inner city food deserts.

In December 2011, I visited Dr. Laurie Hartman, Director of Advanced Practice Nursing at the University of Michigan Hospital System and Clinical Assistant Professor at the School of Nursing. While there, I learned that the demand for acute care nurse practitioners (ACNPs) is on the rise as seniors live longer as a result of advances in medical care. Laurie works constantly to build relationships between the hospital NP staff and the School of Nursing faculty by fostering critical connections between the two organizations. She also encourages her APNs to keep up-to-date on regulations at the state and national levels. From Laurie, I learned about the leadership challenges she faces as she attempts to expand productive interactions between the clinical and the academic. I also learned that a shared governance structure cannot be built in six months but rather requires leadership across departments, ongoing collaboration between healthcare providers, and the fostering of trust.

In March 2011, I had the opportunity to visit Sandra Ryan, Chief Nurse Practitioner Officer for Take Care Health Systems (TCHS) in Conshohocken, Pennsylvania. Sandra oversees clinical and business operations for retail clinics in select Walgreens stores. Convenient care clinics (CCCs) for children, adults, and seniors offer a lower cost alternative to physician-provided services. More than one in three consumers has an interest in visiting a retail clinic, with interest especially high among baby boomers and young adults. At retail clinics, a focus on quality, compassionate, patient-centered care provided by NPs helps keep costs under control and increases patient satisfaction. I learned the value of this lower cost alternative to physician-provided care, especially during the cold and flu season, the allergy season, and for school physicals. I also learned that TCHS believes strongly that collaboration among healthcare professionals is the key to better patient outcomes and provider satisfaction.

During that same March trip, I met up with Dr. Wendy Grube, Director of the Nurse Practitioner Program at the University of Pennsylvania. Twice a year, Wendy takes NP and midwifery students to the Webster County Memorial Hospital in Webster Springs, West Virginia, to conduct breast and cervical cancer screenings for women in the surrounding mountain regions. She wants to tap local communication channels to disseminate accurate cancer information and hopes to use those channels to better understand the sociocultural influences affecting reproductive healthcare and screening practices in the area. Southern women tell each other stories about illness and recovery to reach an understanding about cancer and cope with their own or a loved one's illness. The goal of programs like Wendy's is to increase cancer education throughout Appalachia and to reinforce that caring healthcare providers can be important sources of accurate information in the fight against this feared disease.

In March 2012, I met with Dottie Deremo and Roxanne Roberts from Hospice of Michigan (HOM) in Detroit. Seniors now make up 13 percent of the U.S. population. With the nation growing older, palliative care and hospice services have important roles to play in preparing older adults to maintain control over their lives and face death with dignity. Dottie and Roxanne explained how

HOM puts the patient and his or her family at the center of care planning and, by working closely with physicians and caregivers, provides comprehensive and compassionate care for individuals nearing the end of life. Both Dottie and Roxanne stressed that the patient's wishes are to be respected, even if family members press for more aggressive care. I learned that many patients prefer to die in the comfort of their home, surrounded by family and friends. Hospice care makes this possible by providing pain, psychological, and spiritual support and helping families understand how they can most effectively support their loved one in the final months of life.

In November 2012, I visited Dr. Lisa Chism, who is affiliated with Karmanos Cancer Center in Detroit, Michigan. Lisa currently practices in a multidisciplinary breast center at Karmanos Cancer Institute and is also a Certified Menopause Practitioner and a member of the Patient Education Committee for the North American Menopause Society. She was recently honored as a fellow of the American Academy of Nurse Practitioners and has been involved with the Women's Wellness Clinic in Farmington Hills, Michigan. Lisa's goals are to provide guidance, support, and screenings for women with a history of breast cancer and also to conduct extensive workshops on menopause. I also came to appreciate how she has become such an advocate for the Doctor of Nursing Practice program, about which she has written a book, *The Doctor of Nursing Practice: A Guidebook for Role Development and Professional Issues* (2009, updated in 2013).

In December 2012, I had the immense pleasure of meeting two certified registered nurse anesthetists, Dr. Rosalyn Harrison and Dr. Michael Dosch, both of whom provided me with a unique look into the world of a CRNA. Roz works at St. John Macomb Hospital in Warren, Michigan, where she collaborates with colleagues to ensure that the anesthesia choice and dose are on target, gives patients a warm blanket, solicits questions from the patient and family members, works with the surgeon on the plan of care, and collaborates with physicians, the chief anesthetist, and nurses in the operating room. Mike has been working at Oakwood Hospital and Medical Center in Dearborn, Michigan, for the past eight years. He explained that, as a safety measure, before every surgery everyone on the team introduces each other, takes time to breathe and remind each other that there are certain red lines they cannot cross because doing so would not be safe for the patient. I learned from these two providers that working as a CRNA in a hospital requires patience, appreciation, cooperation, and a deep faith in what others are doing.

Meeting and talking with these dedicated professionals has stoked an enduring appreciation for all those who have committed themselves to expanding their education and clinical skills as advanced practice nurses. I truly believe that they are the future of healthcare in the 21st century. I offer these dedicated individuals my heartfelt support as they develop and hone their approaches to practice—while continuing to search for the best ways to effectively support all of their patients.

TABLE OF CONTENTS

CHAPTER 1

Expanding the Nurse Practitioner Ranks to Meet the Demands for Care

The Patient Protection and Affordable Care Act (PPACA) of 2010 will provide access to health insurance coverage to 32 million previously uninsured people by 2014. The PPACA has sparked a national dialogue, but it fails to address the critical issue: Americans are suffering not only from a lack of health *coverage*, but from a lack of health *care* as well.

Health insurance spending has increased dramatically in recent years. In the first decade of the twenty-first century, premiums for employer-provided health insurance for the average family almost doubled: from $6,800 in 2000 to $12,700 in 2008. Increases of that magnitude erode employers' profits, shunt greater cost burdens onto employees, and ultimately result in reductions in coverage.[1] Without workplace health insurance, Americans struggle to find coverage or simply do without.

Skyrocketing medical costs take a huge toll on America's fiscal health. Since 1994, the per-person cost of healthcare has increased at more than twice the rate of inflation. Rising prescription drug costs, poor outpatient care, unnecessary medical procedures, and fast-rising insurance premiums burden federal and state governments, businesses, and families. Richard Bohmer[2] estimates that the American healthcare system squanders 50 percent of its financial resources through unnecessary bureaucracy, duplicate tests, and other wasteful spending.

Between 2005 and 2007, 72 million adults and children and 7 million seniors experienced difficulties paying their medical bills, bringing the total to 79 million adults with medical debt. .[3] The

Commonwealth Fund[4] found that adults without health insurance or who have gaps in their coverage regularly go without care, which leads to higher medical costs in the future. 61 percent of adults with steep health care bills had health insurance at the time when care was provided. Families struggling to pay off accumulated medical debt are particularly hard hit; often sacrificing health insurance and healthcare visits in their attempts to meet their financial obligations.

Most private health insurance will continue to be offered through employers, whether or not the PPACA is implemented as written. Even so, our healthcare system is inadequately prepared to meet the demands of the millions more Americans who will become insured under full enactment of the PPACA. The aging of our society presents a particular challenge to our already overburdened healthcare system. There are now more Americans aged 65 and older than at any other time in U.S. history.[5] Seniors are especially in need of quality, affordable care. Without change, our healthcare system will not be able to handle the burgeoning population of seniors with high expectations and sometimes frustrating and often-multidimensional medical problems.

A Diminishing Supply of Primary Care Physicians

The 32 million newly covered lives will place unprecedented demand on medical offices, clinics, and hospitals. Couple that with an already diminishing supply of primary care physicians. The American Academy of Family Physicians predicts a shortfall of 40,000 primary care providers by 2020.[6] Medical students increasingly are choosing careers in high-status, higher-paying specialties.[7] The scope of practice for many primary care doctors is diminishing, often restricted to the ongoing care of patients suffering from chronic conditions such as diabetes, obesity, and hypertension; short acute episodes of viral infections; or yearly examinations. The salary differential between PCPs and specialists is substantial: about $250,000 for an internist, compared with $351,000 for a dermatologist and about $694,000 for a neurosurgeon. Medical students cannot pay off their school bills on fees from a career as a primary care physician.

Since Massachusetts's passage of healthcare reform in 2006, nearly 96 percent of the state's residents have health insurance, but the waiting time to see a primary care physician can be up to ninety days.[8] Only 65 percent of adult patients report having access to a personal physician, and three out of every four sick adults cannot get a same-day appointment without going to the emergency room (ER).[9] Forty percent of patients cannot get advice from their physician by phone during regular business hours, and 60 percent cannot get care at night, on weekends, or on holidays without going to the ER.

Shifting Primary Care Provision to NPs and PAs

One way to address this primary care bottleneck is to look at healthcare comprehensively—and to expand the role of advanced practice provider. When millions of new patients enter the healthcare system, many routine care needs *will have to be* met by nurse practitioners (NPs) and physician assistants (PAs). Researchers are exploring the shift of primary care from physicians to NPs and PAs as a means to contain costs and increase access.[10] They are a critical component in the overall solution to our healthcare troubles; together they can help resolve the mounting physician shortage, care for an aging population, and work with chronic illnesses such as diabetes, asthma, coronary heart disease, and bronchitis.

New models for providing effective primary and chronic disease management make use of interdisciplinary teams of clinicians and physicians providing integrated care. These care models, called medical homes or integrated medical groups, have been shown to improve care quality and patient satisfaction while reducing costs at the Veterans Administration Health System, Geisinger Health System, and Kaiser Permanente.[11] In primary care, NPs and PAs perform many of the same tasks as family physicians, including the routine management of chronic diseases. Research suggests that between 25 and 70 percent of care currently handled by physicians can be moved to NPs and PAs.[12]

Many states have expanded or are considering expanding the authority of NPs to work collaboratively with physicians to provide care for the expected patient influx.[13] Between 1995 and 2006, primary care residency programs declined by 3 percent, yet NP programs grew at a rate of 61 percent.[14]

Not only does NP-provided care have the potential to reduce costs, and these providers are able to deliver high-quality care. Utilizing NPs to their fullest potential to treat conditions that traditionally have been handled by primary care physicians will enable physicians and specialists to focus on the more complex cases.[15] Under this forward-looking healthcare model, when patients enter the practice, caregivers will engage with them and actively listen to determine their needs and goals. Caregivers will then develop a customized care plan for each patient, which should help limit diagnostic imaging and medication orders to those that are appropriate for the situation.

The Expansion of Integrated Medical Groups

Healthcare of the future will be based in large part on a foundation of primary care coordinated through patient-centered, integrated medical groups (IMGs). An important characteristic of IMGs is their centralized organizational structure, in which the physicians are employees or partners. IMGs integrate multiple medical specialties into one large system to provide one-stop, high-quality, low-cost healthcare to patients with all kinds of conditions. The IMG concept depends on a sound foundation of primary care provided by both physicians and advanced practice providers such as NPs and PAs.

Donald Berwick[16] states that *"[i]mproving the U.S. health care system requires simultaneous pursuit of three aims: improving the experience of care, improving the health of populations, and reducing the per capita costs of health care."* Physicians, NPs, PAs, and clinical staff need to require that their patients continually become better informed about their health status and how to best manage their own health. Patients struggling with chronic conditions need an advanced practice provider to help them establish an individualized plan, to help them interpret that care plan, and to act as an advocate for their rights. Advanced practice providers can establish long-term relationships with their patients, help them navigate their way through hosptials and specialists and connect them with community resources. Patients are happy with their care and there are no compromises in quality.

How the NP Role Complements the New Healthcare Models

The NP role was created to provide longer patient consultations and to offer patient education, both of which improve care quality and complement physician care. One study, "Advanced Practice Nurse Outcomes 1990–2008: A Systematic Review,"[17] found that patient outcomes provided by nurse practitioners, nurse midwives, and acute care nurses in collaboration with physicians were similar, if not better, than care provided by physicians alone. U.S. healthcare professionals need to move forward with evidence-based and collaborative care models. A smooth-running health system includes multiple providers actively communicating with each other and accountable for delivering fully coordinated care that is individualized for each patient.

Duke University Medical System's clinic for treating congestive heart failure exemplifies this type of integrated care. It places patients in the care of one of two distinct teams. The first unit focuses on uncomplicated cases and is staffed by NPs who apply standard protocols to manage patients. These patients usually respond to treatment and move forward with their care as expected. The second unit focuses on more complicated cases and is staffed by cardiologists. The cardiologists use a wide variety of tests, therapies, and customized procedures to address these more involved and challenging cases. Properly transferring patients from the first unit to the second requires ongoing open communication between the NPs and the cardiologists. Staff of the two units discuss cases and determine together when it is necessary to move patients from one unit to the other. All patients receive ongoing, reliable care in a supportive environment; those with complications receive specialized treatment from physicians who are free to focus on their specific needs.

The *Future of Nursing* Report:
Observations on Practice

The 2010 Institute of Medicine report, *The Future of Nursing: Leading Change, Advancing Health*,[18] has achieved landmark status for its influence on national conversations about nursing practice. The report advocates four main points:

1. **Nurses should practice to the full extent of their education and training.** Their ability to do so involves removing scope of practice laws and assumes that nurses understand their limitations and reach out to physicians when necessary. Physicians and nurses need to build the trust and positive energy that enhances good relationships and reduce the negative energy that impedes trust.

2. **Nurses should achieve higher levels of education and training through an improved education system that promotes seamless academic progression.** In universities across America, NP enrollment is steadily increasing and salaries for those with NP credentials are going up. However, within the next ten years, half of the nursing faculty will reach retirement. Universities must answer the call and figure out ways to step up training for NPs.

3. **Nurses should be full partners with physicians and other health professionals in redesigning healthcare in the**

United States. The vision of what constitutes primary care in America and where it is headed remains shortsighted. Successful healthcare reform will require that physicians and nurses work together within a medical home model.

4. **Effective workforce planning and policy making require better data collection and a better information infrastructure.** Physicians, nurses, and other healthcare providers need to lead the way in building a system for collecting and analyzing inter-professional healthcare data. With the use of EMR technology, patients' health data, genetic makeup, and other personal information can be made available to help predict the health challenges they may face.

Impediments to Using NPs in Primary Care

In general, NPs and primary care physicians perform many of the same functions (e.g., order tests, diagnose and treat illness, prescribe medications, and make referrals to specialists). Although physician practice is fairly uniform across the states, the laws that define NP scope of practice vary significantly from state to state. Given the growing shortage of primary care doctors, some physician organizations are acknowledging that they will need the assistance of NPs in the future.[19]

There remain some significant impediments to using NPs in primary care.

1. **State laws that articulate prescriptive authority:** Twenty-eight states and Washington, D.C., currently grant prescriptive authority to NPs. Ideally, for both professional consistency and patient benefit, the remaining states would join together in authorizing NPs to prescribe. In states where NPs have greater levels of prescriptive authority, the quality of care remains the same, and patient satisfaction

goes up. Scope of practice, relationship with the physician, and liability are also defined by the states and differ from state to state.

2. **Disparate reimbursement policies:**[20] NPs are typically reimbursed at 85 percent of the standard physician rate. To ensure adequate patient access to their provider of choice and to acknowledge the role NPs already play in healthcare, payer policies should reimburse NPs and physicians equitably.

3. **Tensions between physicians, NPs, and PAs:**[21] "Collaboration" between NPs, PAs, and physicians can take many forms and is governed by state law and regulation. Reframing the regulatory restrictions across the United States into an evidence-based vision with a patient safety orientation should be a prime goal for NPs. Clinicians and patients will both benefit from a truly collaborative (rather than a managerial) relationship between NPs and physicians.

Much is left to do to reinvigorate American healthcare. The enigma of how the NP fits into the evolving healthcare system will be solved through collaboration, decreasing practice barriers, and utilizing these professionals to their fullest potential. Other areas that need attention include resolving disparities in pay, granting prescriptive authority, learning to work within integrative teams, defining the roles and responsibilities of the various healthcare professionals, improving metrics that define care standards, investing in information technologies that support primary care centers, and promoting stronger ties between academic medical systems, hospitals, and primary care centers.

NPs look to advance in their own role and within the nursing profession. They do not claim, nor do they aspire, to be physicians.

Barbara Redman, dean of the college of nursing at Detroit's Wayne State University[22], has noted, *"It is clear that the U.S. does not have an adequate primary care workforce. We have too many specialists and need a much larger percentage of the workforce for primary care."* In the best of worlds, healthcare reform will work: Politicians will make efforts to increase funding to meet patient demand, private and government payment sources will increase reimbursements to those providing the care, and the use of medical homes and telemedicine technology will increase, reducing primary care costs and improving care quality. It is in this world that NPs and PAs will find their rightful place working alongside physicians for the betterment of all of their patients.

Growing NP/PA Workforce Challenges
Size of Physician Workforce

Today there are about 140,000 NPs and 83,000 PAs in the current U.S. NP/PA workforce—making the NP/PA group 75 percent the size of the physician group. The NP and PA fields show consistent professional growth and expansion in both primary care and specialty settings, even in these economically challenging times. *U.S. News and World Report,* Monster.com, and CNN/*Money* have ranked NP and PA among the top 10 careers.[23] The U.S. Bureau of Labor Statistics predicts that from 2008 to 2018, there will be a 23 percent increase in overall nursing jobs and a 41 percent increase in PA jobs.[24]

NPs and PAs are an important part of the solution to our U.S. healthcare challenges, which include physician shortages; an increasing aging population; and chronic illnesses like diabetes, cancer, asthma, and coronary heart disease, which remain the leading causes of morbidity in our population. Awareness of what NPs and PAs can accomplish in such settings as retail health, acute care, public and private hospitals, rural health, and school-based health clinics is growing. According to Robert Wooten,[25] PA-C, president of the American Academy of Physician Assistants, *"As America changes from a fragmented to an integrated healthcare delivery system, more attention needs to be placed on a cost-effective care model. More PAs and [NPs] must be empowered to deliver care to the full extent of their education and expertise."*

A Remedy for the Healthcare Crisis

Advanced Practice Nursing examines how some outstanding advanced-practice nurses are using their clinical skills and leadership abilities to move the field of advanced-practice nursing forward in a variety of healthcare venues. In its eight case studies, the book offers a field guide to practical action steps that all NPs can immediately put into practice. It also provides compelling examples that should inspire nurses to consider pursuing advanced education and actively promoting their profession. Every chapter is based on research—both original and that of other prominent leadership theorists.

NPs and PAs, working shoulder to shoulder with physicians, can resolve the mounting crisis on the front lines of healthcare. The studies are told by the NPs, in their own voices, and show how in each case NPs are resolving health care issues in as a certified nurse-midwife, providing care for dying patients, conducting breast and cervical cancer screenings for rural women, overseeing retail health clinics, working with school children and their families, building relationships between NPs and the School of Nursing, working collaboratively with physicians and nurses, and treating women with cancer and serving as a menopause practitioner. The case studies in this book show how eight NPs are serving those who might otherwise fail to receive the care they need:

- Joan Slager, a certified nurse-midwife at Bronson Women's Service in Kalamazoo, Michigan, draws on her specialized training in both nursing and midwifery to provide primary healthcare for all women.

- Dottie Deremo, president and CEO of Hospice of Michigan in Detroit, works closely with physicians and caregivers to provide comprehensive and compassionate care for individuals nearing the end of life.

- Wendy Grube, director of the Women's Health Care Nurse Practitioner Program at the University of Pennsylvania in Philadelphia, takes her students to Webster Springs, West Virginia, to conduct breast and cervical cancer screenings for women who would otherwise not receive them.

- Sandra Ryan, the chief nurse practitioner officer for Take Care Health Systems in Conshohocken, Pennsylvania, oversees retail health clinical and operational activities and works closely with Walgreens as chief medical officer.

- Jonnie Hamilton, a nurse practitioner at Marcus Garvey Academy in Detroit, serves as a hands-on care provider for schoolchildren and their families while also educating her patients about healthy life choices and disease prevention.

- Laurie Hartman, an acute care nurse practitioner working with both the University of Michigan Hospital System and the U-M School of Nursing in Ann Arbor, helps build relationships between the hospital's NP staff and the SON faculty.

- Michael Dosch, CRNA and PhD, Oakwood Hospital and Medical Center, and Roz Harrison, CRNA and DNAP, St. John Macomb Hospital working collaboratively with physicians and nurses around safety protocols and patient health. Chapter concludes with getting into a CRNA nursing school.

- Lisa Chism, DNP, currently practices at Karmanos Cancer Institute in Detroit Michigan and is a Certified Menopause Practitioner and has published and presented on the topic of the Doctor of Nursing Practice degree. Chapter concludes with getting into a DNP program.

The book concludes with a passionate plea to use America's primary care workforce more effectively to prevent illnesses, manage chronic diseases, and promote healthy living. Americans deserve the very best that healthcare has to offer. At the conclusion of this book, APNs will take away the following:

- An understanding of the philosophical and research-based model of APN leadership and grasp the fundamental concepts of why good leadership works and how APNs can make the model work for them.

- A list of practical leadership steps at the end of each chapter, actions that require all APNs and PAs take charge and lead others towards better health for all and increased collaboration among all team members.

- Thinking about the requirements for change that each NP or PA needs to consider before taking the plunge that requires each of us to reflect on our paths going forward.

- Best practice advice gleaned from years of working in the business world of manufacturing, banking, insurance, energy, universities and the health industry.

- And most important, a comprehensive field guide of action steps that require little or no budget and no approvals from management but do require commitment to internalize the steps and the discipline to make them happen.

CHAPTER TWO

The Certified Nurse Midwife: Practice Vision, Collaborative Relationships, and Billing Concerns

By definition, a certified nurse-midwife (CNM) is an advanced practice nurse (APN) who has specialized education and training in both nursing and midwifery. CNMs function as primary healthcare providers for pregnant women, most often relatively healthy women, whose pregnancies are considered uncomplicated (not "high risk") and whose babies are not at risk.[1] But CNMs do much more than deliver babies; they address maternity care, promote healthy living, counsel women for family planning and contraceptive use, conduct gynecologic procedures, treat infertility issues, detect and treat breast problems, and address osteoporosis and menopausal concerns.

This chapter relates the experience of a group of midwives who worked with physicians and hospital administration to restructure the OB-GYN services at Bronson Women's Service (BWS) under a midwifery model. Their success in working collaboratively with physicians to provide quality women's healthcare offers a model for those wishing to do the same. BWS stands by its innovative midwife approach to childbirth. Its website[2] summarizes that experience quite well:

Childbirth that's less medical, more natural—and care for women of all ages. Bronson is pleased to offer Michigan's largest midwifery practice and board-certified OB/GYN doctors, too.

BWS has never wavered on its policy. If you are having

a baby, you will see a midwife. If someone comes in and says, "I want to see a doctor," then we will provide them with a list of OB doctors in the area. But we are essentially a midwife service with doctors as backup. Physicians are available for consultation or referrals, depending on the needs of the patients. But essentially midwives and physicians work collaboratively to address women's health concerns.

How Crisis Generated an Opportunity

When four doctors unexpectedly left the OB/GYN practice at Bronson Methodist Hospital (BMH) in Kalamazoo, Michigan, 19 years ago, the practice lacked any qualified physicians to care for the extremely large number of pregnant women seeking services. Because Dr. Silvio Aladjem, the practice's chief of perinatology, and Joan Slager, a certified nurse-midwife, had worked together in a collaborative relationship in the past, Dr. Aladjem suggested to the hospital CEO and Board that BMH consider a midwifery model for its practice. He then contacted Joan, who was practicing midwifery at the nearby Family Health Center of Battle Creek, Michigan, where midwives had created a well-organized and efficient model of women's healthcare delivery. When approached by the BWS regional nurse liaison, Joan and the other midwives at the Family Health Center felt confident they could replicate the same model at BWS:

> Joan Slager: *Dr. Aladjem felt that we had a good model for midwifery and could add value to the Bronson system. High-risk doctors are not interested in regular births; midwives specialize in normal deliveries. With a practice setting and patient population already in place and an accredited hospital [Bronson Methodist], we sold them on a model of care that would use fewer resources, maintain quality, and get better patient satisfaction.*

Articulating the Midwifery Vision

In its initial stage, the plan was more philosophical than financial. Joan and the midwives with whom she worked articulated a vision of what midwives could do for pregnant women. Focusing specifically on person-hours, BMH only wanted to know how many patients a midwife could see in one day. Because BMH lacked bylaws granting practice privileges to midwives, its staff held multiple meetings to revise the institutional bylaws, create collaborative agreements with physicians, and develop practice guidelines. In addition, Joan and her team of midwives had to educate the BMH attorney and other administrators about midwifery and how such a model would work for pregnant women and within the hospital.

Both Joan and the other midwives quickly learned not to assume that everyone shared their knowledge about midwifery. They had to apply their vision to their new situation. They had to do their homework on what it takes to adapt a midwife practice to the full extent of the applicable laws, including federal and state laws and BMH local bylaws. They had to become familiar with the rules and regulations of the Joint Commission on Accreditation of Healthcare Organizations (JCAHO), now The Joint Commission (TJC). And they had to understand any practice agreements with the physicians with whom they would be collaborating.[3] The midwives and the physicians both needed to learn the importance of keeping senior level executives, office managers, and the hospital board of trustees up-to-date on all rule changes, amendments to practice guidelines, and individualized protocols.

Participants in the new practice had to establish formal guidelines, such as knowing the legal basis for the practice, defining the patient population, defining the scope of practice, and working within the BMH system. The physicians and the midwives of BWS work collaboratively but maintain their mutual independence. Physicians at BWS need to keep an open mind, because midwives do things differently.

After working intensively with key BMH administrators, the health care attorney, and members of the obstetric medical staff,

Joan and the other midwives developed a business plan and a model for a midwife practice. Initially, the contract and model were based on what was in place at the Family Health Center of Battle Creek. While these midwives intended to return to Battle Creek, they ended up staying at BWS and creating a new model based on their evolving vision of midwifery care. That model involves providing care for women during their pregnancies, labor, and the birthing process; working with them as they learn to care for their newborns during their hospital stay and when they return. But CNMs go beyond caring for pregnant women to provide well-woman care related to reproductive health, annual gynecologic exams, family planning, and menopausal care.

How CNMs Prepare Patients for the Birth Experience

You are a midwife, assisting at someone else's birth. Do good without show or fuss. If you must take the lead, lead so the mother is helped, yet still free and in charge. When the baby is born, the mother will rightly say: "We did it ourselves!

—from the Tao Te Ching

CNMs foster a high-touch personal environment that comforts women at all stages of pregnancy. Midwives gain their patients' trust and excel at really listening to their patients' concerns and offering guidance about what to expect from the labor experience. CNMs tend to have longer consultations with their patients and to provide them with more information than doctors do.

CNMs care about their patients' physical and emotional health. They ask mothers-to-be questions about their preparations for the birth of their child or children, counsel them in their choice of breast- or bottle-feeding, and encourage them to eat nutritious meals. They also want clients to recognize the changes that are going on in their bodies, to attend a birthing class, and to know what to do before they go into labor. They encourage women to read pamphlets and books on pregnancy and to write down the lessons learned. All this and more is a part of the education and support midwives offer women approaching the miracle of the birthing process. Midwives acknowledge that birthing a child hurts, but assure women that all will be forgotten in the rush of love when they hold their tiny babies.

The simple act of sitting and maintaining eye contact with a patient boosts the patient's feelings of trust and promotes a more enduring relationship. When a CNM sits when seeing a patient, the patient perceives the interaction to be three times longer than when the CNM stands. However, real sharing comes when both the midwife and the client exchange true experiences and are present in the moment.[4] But how do midwives find the time for true sharing while attending to all the tasks leading up to the birth of a baby? Often it is the client's last question, just as the midwife is leaving the room, that reveals the "real" issues—and the emotions pour out. These situations challenge the midwife to truly listen and to appreciate what the woman is experiencing.

Reassuring the Doubters

The first order of business for the BWS midwives was to dispel the notion among existing staff that they might jeopardize patient safety and welfare. Staff initially feared that the quality of care would decline and their patients would suffer. They believed that the hospital was "giving in" to the midwives' demands. But the midwives took command and convinced the doubters by modeling what they could offer the practice's patients. In meetings with the staff, Joan and her midwives answered questions like these: *"Where did you come from? What is your skill level? How would you manage patients like ours? What will you do when there are patient problems?"*

From "Clinic" to "Private Care" Model

Under the former system at BWS, each incoming patient call was announced over the intercom, and whoever was available picked up the call. This resulted in fragmented care for the caller, and it interrupted other patients' care. With a phone nurse in place under the new system, women could call and ask questions about their bodies and what was happening to them. Hearing a nurse with a friendly voice on the other end of the phone meant a lot to the women calling in and immediately established empathy. There were questions about swollen ankles, hemorrhoids, and the use of medications. After this system was established, the hospital dramatically decreased its emergency room visits, saving significant costs.

The BWS practice originally had no dedicated appointment times. The first available physician saw women in the order in which they checked in. Women who came to the practice often brought a lunch because they never knew when they would be seen. The midwives changed that practice, assigning callers regular appointment times at specific times during the day. They asked patients to honor their appointment times and told them that if they could not show up on time, they would have to reschedule. Having a defined schedule helps both clients and staff nurses manage their time effectively.

Joan and her seven midwives changed the way women were treated at BWS to more of a private care model. Instead of being a place where women went if they had no insurance, now patients could choose their healthcare providers. Respect for clients was key. BWS helped paint the waiting room, provided wooden and fabric chairs, and hung new pictures. The waiting rooms were cleaned and provisioned with new clinic tables and equipment. With the practice environment looking better, clients waiting for their scheduled appointments felt happier. BWS clients now had an environment every bit as good as that found in a private care model.

How the Midwife Model Decreases C-Section Rates

Midwives do whatever it takes to allow healthy mothers to have their babies normally. Midwives are dedicated to providing direct, one-on-one care by getting women out of bed and walking. When the midwife on call goes off shift, another midwife immediately takes over, providing continuity of care and responsibility.

Joan Slager: *I wasn't interested in physicians who wanted to do normal births; we [midwives] do normal births. [At BWS] you get a doctor if you need a C-section, if you are having twins, have hypertension, or have diabetes. If you have any of these conditions, you will be seen by a doctor but will be attended by a midwife during delivery.*

Only after the attending midwife has consulted appropriately with the labor nurse and the obstetrician and after she has exhausted all approaches available to her within her scope of practice is the patient referred for a potential Cesarean delivery (C-section). Only after all quality and safety standards are followed and the midwife makes all the proper referrals does the obstetrician take over and the C-section proceed.

Susan Imanse: *The role of the labor nurse is always supportive; she walks with the woman, holds hands during the bad parts of labor, plays music, or just sits and talks. The role of the midwife and the labor nurse often overlap. With multiple women giving birth, the midwife cannot be with each one all the time. Instead, the labor nurse, the midwife, and the woman form a team, with one goal: the safe birth of the child or children. The midwife understands the "why," and the labor nurse makes it happen.*

It's a different scenario when a physician is involved: Often, when a physician comes into the operating room, he or she demands control.

Susan Imanse: *Physicians change the energy in the room. When I am in the labor room getting the woman ready for delivery and the physician comes in, now the patient has to push differently. Now we are focusing on the physician, not the mother, and my job is to focus on the physician only. With a midwife, the focus remains on the woman.*

In 2009, rates for C-section deliveries in America climbed to 34 percent, hitting an all-time high.[5] Groups such as the World Health Organization argue that the rate should be about 15 percent. There are no data showing that higher rates improve outcomes, yet C-sections continue to climb higher.

Within three months of the midwives' arrival at BWS, the C-section rate at the practice dropped from 30 percent to 14 percent; more important, the patient satisfaction rate dramatically improved. (When it "slipped" to 98 percent, the midwives made it a point to address patient concerns.) More significantly, as the rate of C-sections decreased, so did costs and overhead. Obviously, if BWS can show lower C-section rates with the use of midwives, insurance companies will take note and reimburse accordingly.

Profile of the Collaborating Physicians at BSW

They should be doing childbirth surgery all day, every day, when needed. They should not be doing normal births, because they're not trained in it. They have no idea how to do it.

—Elan Vital McAllister, president,
New York's Choices in Childbirth

The connection between the midwife and the collaborating physician opens conversations about scope of practice, appropriate protocols, and the need to document collaborative agreements. Both staff at BSW and the incoming midwives came to understand that good communication spawns trust and failed communication erodes it. When this was fully understood, BWS hired its first physician. The practice was growing rapidly.

Although the practice formerly was 99 percent Medicaid recipients, nurses in Labor and Delivery and other privately insured women in the community began to come to the practice to deliver their babies. As demand for services increased, BWS hired another physician. The physicians came to understand that the practice was a nurse-run midwifery service, not one run by physicians; it does not have a residency program because residents take patients away from the midwives. The practice hired only physicians who could work collaboratively with the midwives.

BWS did not hire physicians who had just completed their medical rotations. Rather, the practice hired those who had done the required births and who were really into gynecologic procedures. BWS only took physicians who had been in practice for a number of years and who, because of the breadth of their clinical and surgical experience, preferred not to handle uncomplicated normal births. BWS physicians are kept busy doing intricate surgeries and complicated procedures and dealing with high-risk pregnancies—in other words, working to the level of their abilities as capable and skilled physicians. This allows the physicians to generate significant amounts of revenue, which keeps them happy and the midwives even happier.

Dr. Zylkia Rodriguez, BWS medical director, describes her search for a physician:

> Dr. Rodriguez: *When we lost one of the physicians four or five years ago, I had to interview so many physicians before making a new selection. First of all they needed to understand that 50 percent of the patients are indigent or have no insurance. Plus, regular obstetrics won't happen, because the midwives do the normal births.* [Many of the interviewees] *said,* "OK, this is not for me." *We finally found someone, and he never wants to leave.*

Serving a Broad Patient Base with Respect

One way to measure a particular doctor's openness and attitude toward women in general is simply to ask about the doctor's opinion of midwifery.

—Marsden Wagner,

The BWS practice developed a philosophy that emphasizes partnerships between midwives and physicians. The midwives did

21

not want to work within a find-it/fix-it disease-based model, which marks the medical approach to pregnancy and childbirth.

BWS takes patients who have not had prenatal care, no matter how far along in their pregnancies they are. If a patient comes to the practice at 26 weeks with an infection, she is encouraged to follow up. If another comes in at term and has her baby at BWS, the midwives can still handle the situation. They do not make judgments about why the patient did or did not receive prenatal care; they just take care of her. Chastising patients for not getting prenatal care does not work; finding out why they have failed to seek out care helps them. Initially, patients without insurance do not understand that they will not end up with a massive bill. The midwives encourage women to get the tests, the ultrasounds, and the lab work they need.

If a patient feels bad about having Medicaid coverage and believes the midwives are judging her, she might not return to the practice for follow-up. If she perceives that the midwives have a different set of rules for her than for patients with private insurance, that may well change her willingness to get treatment. Some women have been told all of their lives that because of their poverty, their race, or their religion, they do not matter. BWS, however, works with people from all cultures and treats everyone equally, with respect. This approach has always been a part of BWS's values.

Building Partnerships with Private-Practice Physicians

The private physicians practicing near BWS could have been the midwives worst enemies. However, due to the midwives' efforts at professional collaboration, that has not been the case. The midwives have learned that effective partnerships require both mutual goals and active team building.[6] They have also learned to make use of the physicians' influence and referral base. Formerly, private-practice physicians simply provided backup coverage; now they call the midwives to sit with their patients while they handle other emergencies—and the midwives watch their patients as a professional courtesy. Mutual trust is the very foundation of collaboration. Trust spawns successful relationships.

Joan Slager: *When we have quarterly medical staff breakfasts, I could sit with the other nurse practitioners, but I don't. I sit with the cardiologists and the trauma surgeons. I introduce myself and tell them what I do, how fun my job is, and some of the rewarding things I do. It is all about selling yourself and your profession.*

Having privileges in a hospital means that the midwives have to take their turn at "no-doc" patients. The midwives take unassigned OB patients, those who come to the hospital without prenatal care, those who are in town on vacation or attending a wedding or funeral, and those who otherwise have no doctor. The midwives step up and do what the physicians are reluctant to do. That is something that the staff physicians have come to value.

Joan Slager: *The midwives add value to the organization and their practice by seeing patients no one else wants to see and offering to provide care that meets the needs of these vulnerable patient populations.*

By caring for patients in need, the midwives have increased their value in the community and to the practice. Because the private physicians recognize the midwives' value, the physicians have become advocates for them, and the midwives are happy to let the physicians support their program model. Physicians may offer high-tech solutions, but midwives offer high-touch solutions.

Each midwife needs to ask herself: *"What niche do I have? What opportunities can I seize that no one else is handling? What can I do that nobody else can or wants to do?"* Even more important, midwives need to make use of physicians' influence and reputation. Physicians willing to collaborate with midwives serve as a source of referrals. Midwives can provide referrals of their own, sending women needing an obstetrician for tubal ligations, ablations, or hysterectomies. That way, everyone is happy.

> Joan Slager: *If you are going to command respect at a meeting or at the country club, you have to see yourself as a member of the team—equal, but different. I may say that I am a midwife and that I am proud of my status. I do not work for doctors; I work with doctors. You have to convey a basic understanding of what you do. Don't apologize for your role—everyone has his or her role.*

Physician Respect for the Midwife Model

The whole point of women-centered birth is the knowledge that a woman is the birth power source. She may need, and deserve, help, but in essence, she always had, currently has, and will have the power.

—Heather McCue
Practicing doula since 2001

Over the years, the physicians have learned that they need to intervene in midwife-provided patient care less and less frequently. They might not value the high-touch care or the level of active patient management midwives provide, but they have learned to respect the professional collaboration they receive from the midwives. The more midwives keep the physicians updated, the more comfortable the physicians feel.

> Mary Alice Martin: *I have never worked in a place where we are so very well respected. We do a lot of high-risk pregnancies, and I will call one of the consulting physicians in Labor and Delivery with my concerns: "I am not sure of the situation and want you to come and check things out." They come because they really believe in you.*

The relationship between the physicians and the midwives has evolved to the point where all the physicians want to hear from the midwives is whether there is a deviation from the norm. Building that kind of trust takes time, of course. There is a proving period, where the midwives must demonstrate to the physicians what they can do. For example, the midwives initially had to notify the physicians whenever a woman was put on Pitocin. Later the physicians decided that they did not want to be called about such things. They said, *"You know what you are doing, and it is OK with us."*

A Holistic View of Pregnancy and Women's Health

The nursing model of pregnancy and birth is very different from the medical model, especially when comparing a midwife with an obstetrician. The nursing model looks at pregnancy holistically. The nurses understand what women bring to the birth experience and how well they are looking after their own health and well-being. Physicians do try to understand, but they focus more on changes to the body during pregnancy and whether a vaginal delivery or a C-section is necessary. Physicians want control, while midwives see childbirth as a "normal" experience. Neither view is wrong; the two are just different.

Nurse-midwives form more of a partnership with their patients. Midwives understand that women need to have power over their bodies. They review the goals of the pregnancy: *"What does this woman want to achieve at the birth of her child? What about after the birth of the child?"* Midwives focus on giving women information about their changing bodies, empowering them to make their own decisions, and letting them direct their own birthing experience, within safety standards. With a midwife, the locus of control stays with the woman; with a physician, the locus of control remains with the physician.

Each woman needs to walk out of the birth experience feeling a sense of accomplishment:

Susan Imanse: *I don't care if they remember my name; I just want them to feel proud about delivering their baby. Each woman needs to own her birth experience and deliver her baby in her own way. So many times I have seen women feel defeated, like they could not do it. With good training, I can prepare these women so that they do have control of their own bodies. They can do this.*

Benefits of the Midwife Model for Physicians

After working with midwives for twelve years, Dr. Rodriguez has developed a very collaborative approach for how she and the midwives handle patients. With the midwives in place, she and the other BWS physicians no longer have to "labor-sit"; instead, they can be in the operating rooms doing surgery or procedures. Because of the midwife services, physicians are not on call as frequently. They do not have to stay up all night with women in labor, then turn around and do surgeries all day. When a midwife reaches an impasse and needs the expertise of a physician, one will be there fresh and available, and physicians can also be there with patients who still want an obstetrician.

Dr. Rodriguez: *I have been at Bronson since 1992. Previously, I worked in a private practice and was always supportive of midwives. I trained with midlevel providers for a long time and enjoyed the working relationship. Having midwives on call every night allows the attending physicians to focus on other health concerns beyond normal pregnancies. Midwives can do normal deliveries, allowing me to focus on high-risk and gynecologic treatments, which are my passion. It is a win-win situation and has put a different spin on how I do medicine. Midwives do routine well, and I can focus more on the high-risk patients.*

Handling Disagreements over Patient Management

Occasionally disagreements develop over patient care, and tempers flare. The midwives make it a point that they do not want to get between two physicians or between a physician and a midwife. Patient management protocol discussions must be in the form of a dialogue. Often when the physicians hear the midwives' rationale for patient management, they understand and agree.

Mary Alice Martin: *If* [a physician] *comes up and starts telling me what to do, I will just say, "Hey, just go ahead and take her. I am not here to follow your plan." Then the physician will say, "Well, maybe you do know what you are doing."*

Dr. Rodriguez and Joan Slager process conflicts and recreate the events leading up to the conflict, but they have one rule, *"We let physicians evaluate physicians and midwives evaluate midwives."* Issues can arise between physicians and midwives because they are trained differently. Even staff physicians do procedures in different ways. Thorough discussion can wash away differences of opinion, and the "right" way will eventually emerge. Turf battles are not necessary when midwives are clear about what they want to do and physicians are clear about what they want to do. Appreciation and dialogue help iron out the differences.

Knowing Your Limits

There are situations when the midwives feel the need for a doctor to evaluate the patient because they believe that they have reached the extent of their skill set and want additional help.

Mary Alice Martin: *The physician might say, "You can handle this," and I might say, "No, I can't." The physicians know when I have gotten to the point where labor is not progressing very far. They accept my call for help. Before, they would conduct their own examination; now they do not. I tell them what the vaginal exam is like, the status of the baby, and how long labor has lasted. They go in and talk to the patient. "Hello, I am doctor so-and-so, and I am going to be doing your C-section."*

The physicians respect us. I have done a number of breech deliveries, and many of the doctors have never done a breech delivery. If I am in the hospital and some feet are hanging out of the vagina, they will say, "Come and stay with me for this delivery."

Even though everyone should know his or her limits, sometimes that line is not clear. This applies to both midwives and physicians. Therefore, the midwife needs to have the confidence to communicate her position. Each midwife needs to ask herself if she should have called the physician earlier. At other times, the physician may wonder why the midwife called him or her in so soon. The physician might feel that another midwife could have handled the problem. But this particular midwife might not have the expertise or self-confidence to handle the situation.

The same is true of physicians. The maternal-fetal physicians say that some physicians call about everything and some do not call at all. Some physicians could step a little closer to the edge but do not choose to because of the risk. Others could have their feet and most of their body hanging off the edge and will not call, when clearly it would have been prudent to ask for help earlier.

Both midwives and doctors have learned that experience is important and that the opportunity to learn from doctors with greater skills creates better midwives. The doctors have learned to understand that when a midwife calls them for help, she has done everything possible and the situation has gone beyond the point where she feels comfortable handling it. The midwife is recognizing the need for the next level of expertise.

Midwives Expanding Their Scope of Care

When a physician leaves, can the midwives do more? Bronson had four perinatologists when one of them had a heart attack and another had a baby. Down to half, with the physicians directing the care and the midwives following the plan, the two remaining perinatologists began to see more high-risk patients. The physicians taught the midwives how to conduct certain procedures, and the midwives taught the physicians their philosophy of caring. While the midwives continued to take care of normal deliveries, they learned that they could take on some of the high-risk OB-GYN patients as well. The Bronson experience shows that midwives can act as obstetric hospitalists providing dedicated, in-hospital care, thereby easing patient load, fatigue, and on-call obligations.[7]

Conveying Passion for the Work Midwives Do

Joan Slager: *When I talk to hospital administration or the chief financial officer, I want to convey a passion for the work we do. The importance of passion cannot be understated. Take accountability for your own statistics; you cannot depend on others to keep your data. No one is going to do your work. You have to say, "This is the value we bring to this organization."*

There were times when [the administration] wanted to cut our salary. I had to dig out statistics and show bar graphs of C-section rates, patient satisfaction scores, and the money that we had generated. No administrator is going to do all that digging. You have to be able to defend your position and say, "You are not allowed to cut our pay or cut a position."

Working toward Equitable Compensation

Physicians are compensated from their billed revenues. Often with third-party medical providers, services are lumped together into one charge, for example, prenatal care, delivery, and postpartum.

Midwifery productivity is evaluated based on relative value units (RVUs), a system that permits other ways of accounting for productivity. Under the global bill, there is only so much available revenue. When it is allocated, the physicians will want to claim their share. Therefore, the midwives use two different yardsticks in order to maintain collaboration without creating competition. Clarity is important when it comes to these different billing procedures; physicians bill through their revenues and midwives bill through the RVU system.

The midwives work on different procedures, and they can bill for multiple services. Although a patient may come in for a well-woman checkup, it is often because something else is bothering her. When the midwife does the Pap smear, she may find that the patient has a polyp on her cervix. The midwife should be able to bill for the removal of the polyp in addition to the well-woman checkup. The BWS practice averages six to eight triage patients per shift; with this volume midwives should be able to bill separately from the global bill. This is important because BWS needs great statistics to back up its claim that it provides its patients with the best health care services possible.

All midwives must create their own data set and prove their own worth. They should not be afraid to bill outside the global bill in the event they encounter a new clinical condition. They must prove their value by showing how much workload each of them can carry, plus the time they spend in administrative functions and teaching. They must learn how to separate time spent working under a physician from the work of the midwife. They must document the value of midwifery care by charting progress on low C-section rates, normal birth weights, and low neonatal admissions. All of these statistics can be shown to insurance companies to validate cost savings, to encourage them to contract with midwives.

Liability Considerations and the
Need for Regulatory Reforms

Litigation often stems from poor communication, misunderstandings, or poor relationships. Often, despite the best practices, lawsuits happen. A CNM's liability coverage is three or four times higher than a regular nurse practitioner's. Midwife delivery of care requires longer prenatal visits, more communication, and more training. BWS's care philosophy is critical to the overall health of the women it serves. Practice guidelines must be kept up-to-date, and deviations from standard practice should not be tolerated. Midwives must learn when and how to consult physicians, and to document, document, document.

Physicians are equally concerned about legal exposure and liability. It is for that reason that physicians do not want midwives to become independent. Of the 1,300 deliveries at BWS in 2010, the physicians had no idea what went on with most of them. They could not know because they are involved only when the midwives involve them. That is how health care works at BWS.

Although midwives in many states can admit under their own names, those in other states are restricted from doing so. State regulations regarding prescriptive authority vary across the country as well: some states grant prescriptive authority to midwives; others do not. In many states, collaborating physicians are required to supervise CNMs in person at their practice setting for a defined amount of time. In other states, collaboration is more discretionary in scope. However, in states where CNMs have greater levels of prescriptive authority, the quality of care does not deteriorate, and patient satisfaction goes up.

Some midwives must bill under a physician's name for payment; the title of "nurse" holds the midwife captive and limits the midwife's ability to charge under her own name. CNMs are typically reimbursed at 85 percent of the standard physician rate. Where does the remaining 15 percent of revenue go? Physicians might consider the 85 percent rate to be equitable, but CNMs need to get paid at the 100 percent rate. To ensure adequate patient access

31

to their provider of choice and to acknowledge the role CNMs already play in healthcare, payer policies should reimburse CNMs and physicians equally.

There is work to be done in multiple areas, including resolution of disparities in pay, the granting of prescriptive authority, ability to work within integrative teams, definition of the roles and responsibilities of the various healthcare professionals, and improving metrics that define care standards. When CNMs and physicians work together in a combined effort, patient's benefit and healthcare concerns decrease. CNMs must work to establish regulations that reframe the regulatory restrictions across the United States into an evidence-based vision with a patient safety orientation.

One Nurse Leader's Accomplishments

Joan Slager has done so much to promote the value of certified nurse midwives by accomplishing the following:

- She established formal guidelines, such as knowing the legal basis for the practice, defining the patient population, defining the scope of practice with physicians, and working within the BMH system.

- She encouraged all of her midwives to prepare the mothers-to-be to ask questions about the birth of their child or children, read pamphlets, attend a labor class, and exchange their own birth stories.

- She reassured the doubters by modeling behaviors, such as establishing set appointment times and having a defined schedule, that help both clients and staff.

- She decreased the C-section rate from 30 to 14 percent while maintaining or improving patient satisfaction.

- She built partnerships with private physicians by offering to care for their patients while the physicians handled other emergencies.

- She handled patient management protocol discussions through dialogue, with evidence-based practice eventually emerging. She documented the value of midwifery care by improving billing practices, documenting midwifery productivity and its contribution to practice revenue, and charting progress on clinical outcomes.

- She promoted patient access to their provider of choice and worked to implement payer policies that acknowledge the important role of CNMs by reimbursing CNMs and physicians equally.

- She improved billing practices, documenting midwifery productivity and its contribution to practice revenue, and charting progress on clinical outcomes.

- She promoted patient access to their provider of choice and worked to implement payer policies that acknowledge the important role of CNMs by reimbursing CNMs and physicians equally.

Conclusion

CNMs can provide quality care by working collaboratively with physicians. Data from physicians demonstrate that working more than eighteen hours consecutively is the equivalent of having a blood alcohol level of 0.08 percent, the limit for drunk driving. Sleep-impaired physicians may not be making decisions that are in the best interest of the patient. However, physicians working collaboratively with CNMs can provide what is best for both patients and their babies. Midwives are less threatening to women than physicians because they reach out to their clients and offer them hope. A collaborative group of seven midwives, all with different skills, working with a physician seems to offer the greatest advantage to both physician and midwifes. Midwives learn procedures from the physicians, and midwives approach women more globally, helping them to feel more at ease. CNMs work hard to take care of their patients, to respond to their special issues, and to provide them with safe and effective ways to deliver their babies and to take care of their own health.

Actions for Nurse Practitioners

Question for Reflection

Healthcare isn't just about seeing patients; it's also about paying the bills. What billing processes can you put in place to increase your financial viability? Look into what you are earning now, and determine alternative ways to bill in the future. You are in no position to negotiate if you don't know what you are worth. From hospitals and clinics to school settings, billing more increases your value.

Billing Practices

- Learn the meaning of financial and accounting terms used in your practice.
- Analyze current billing practices, and identify ways to increase financial viability.

Example:

Know what you are worth. Learn as much as you can about billing and accounts receivable. Bring in billing specialists to talk to your staff about billing codes. Take steps to understand why some insurance companies pay more and why Medicare rejects some claims. Understand that sometimes you have to work under a physician in order to bill properly. Know your statistics and the evidence-based practices; you cannot argue with fact.

Increasing Financial Strength

- Learn to bill outside of the global bill, utilizing the relative value system (RVU).
- Physicians and nurse practitioners need to be billed at the 100 percent rate.

Example:
Value is not always measured in financial terms. Learn to bill outside of the global bill by utilizing the RVU system. For example, if a patient comes in wanting a well-woman checkup, learn to ask your patient if there is anything else she would like examined. Make sure that both you and your physician understand about working with your patient to bill appropriately and wisely.

Documenting Patient Care

- Become familiar with all federal and state rules and regulations that apply to your practice, including Joint Commission on Accreditation of Healthcare Organizations (JCAHO).
- Keep senior level executives and clinic managers up-to-date on all rule changes, amendments to practice guidelines, and individualized protocols.

Example:
All patient care must thorough and measurable, including all medications. Participants in the new practice had to establish formal guidelines, such as knowing the legal basis for the practice, defining the patient population, defining the scope of practice, and working within the hospital system. Patient care, in the end, is defined by patient outcomes and end-of-shift, week, and year records.

Visionary Leadership

Using a Crisis to Further Your Cause

- Determine a response to a crisis or deep-seated need.
- Use the residency rule of not working over 80 hours to your advantage.

Example:

If you work in a community that has reduced resident hours, walk in and offer to help. "I know you have residents who used to help the attending physician. Now that resident hours are limited, there are some gaps in your coverage." Because of the 80-hour work rule, teaching hospitals have also hired more nurse practitioners. Doors swing open far more readily when you act in response to a crisis than when you just say, "Let me in."

Establishing a Guiding Coalition

- Determine areas of care that are not being addressed.
- Understand your customer and examine that customer's needs.

Example:

Identify people who can support you in your future efforts, and reach out to them for support. When you walk into a meeting, do not sit with the other nurse practitioners but with the cardiologists, OB/GYN physicians, and senior level administrators. Show your passion for your job. If you have an idea to sell, find out the best contact within each group. It may be your regular contact or it may be someone else who in more informed on your topic.

CHAPTER THREE

Hospice and Palliative Care: Relationship Building, End-of-Life Care Choices, and Expanding Availability

As the population of those 65 and older soars, hospice and palliative care are growing in importance and relevance. Seniors now make up 13 percent of the U.S. population,[1] a larger percentage than at any time in our country's history. With the nation growing older, long-term care facilities, hospitals, palliative care, and hospice need to be prepared to help older adults maintain control over their lives and face death with dignity. Hospice care can be ordered for those whose life expectancy is six months or less or for whom there are no remaining treatment options. The goal of hospice care is to help patients live their last days alert, pain free, and surrounded by their loved ones.

Hospice treats the person rather than the disease. It focuses on patients and their families, to help all concerned make the crucial decisions about quality, rather than length, of life. That said, patients and their families are truly the best advocates for determining the type of care they receive and which options are best for their particular condition. But they need to prepare themselves to advocate effectively by reading the medical literature, questioning the sources of the information they are given, continuing to be skeptical, and always asking probing questions of their healthcare providers.[2]

The Story of Hospice of Michigan

Since 1998, Dottie Deremo has led Hospice of Michigan (HOM). As CEO and President, Dottie Deremo provides services to meet the emotional, spiritual, and physical needs of HOM's patients and their families. Prior to joining HOM, she served as chief nursing officer for Henry Ford Hospital and was in charge of patient care services at Hutzel Hospital. She has adopted a vision that puts the patient and family at the center of care planning. Working closely with physicians and caregivers, she and HOM provide comprehensive, compassionate care for individuals nearing the end of life and support to their families. But Dottie goes beyond that calling to embrace a leadership philosophy whose mission is to spread hospice and palliative care throughout the United States.

For example, Dottie, in partnership with Steven Grant, M.D., recently signed a contract to help manage the sickest patients in the Detroit Medical Center's new accountable care organization, Michigan Pioneer ACO. Under the contract, @HOMe Support™ (a subsidiary of HOM) will identify terminally ill patients in Michigan Pioneer ACO who have less than twenty-four months to live and provide physical, social, emotional, and spiritual support services at the patients' homes. This alone will save more than 30 percent in medical costs during those last twenty-four months of care. Dottie and Dr. Grant coordinated their efforts to improve care quality, curb emergency room visits, and cut costs during the last year of life. Instead of being sent to the emergency room, participating Medicare patients will be given a phone number to call @HOMe Support™'s nurse call center to coordinate care right at the home and receive services at home as needed.

Founded in 1980, HOM was the State of Michigan's first hospice program. Serving fifty-six counties in the Lower Peninsula of Michigan, HOM covers a large geographical area with an even larger patient population base. HOM is a nonprofit, community-based organization with a defined mission of serving all who need and seek care, regardless of age, diagnosis, or ability to pay. HOM annually raises $4 million to cover the cost of care for the uninsured and underinsured and creates innovative programs that advance end-of-life care. Through its research and education arm, the Maggie Allesee Center for Quality of Life Innovation, HOM provides education programs for physicians, nurses, social workers, aides, and the community and applies research outcomes to improve care and enhance quality of life for patients, families, and the teams that support them.[3]

Hospice of Michigan: In Its Own Words[4]

Hospice of Michigan provides services to meet the emotional, spiritual and physical needs of our patients and their families. Hospice puts the family and patient at the center of care planning, and by working closely with physicians and caregivers, provides comprehensive, compassionate care for individuals nearing the end of life.

Our services include:

- Pain and symptom management.
- Emotional and spiritual support.
- Home health aides and trained volunteers.
- Respite for family caregivers.
- Medications, equipment and supplies.
- Grief support for loved ones.
- In the home.
- In the hospital.
- In the long-term care setting.

Hospice of Michigan's Vision, Mission, and Values[5]

Vision

Innovate end-of-life care in Michigan

Role-model the way for America

Mission

Ensure quality of life, comfort, and peace for our patients; provide support for their loved ones during their end-of-life experience

Serve everyone in our communities who needs and seeks our care; strive to improve the state of comfort care

Building Relationships with Patients, Hospitals, and Nursing Homes

Because of its vision and function, hospice is and always will be a relationship business. Hospice has always been about relationships with patients, but HOM recognizes that it must also build relationships with hospitals, nursing homes, and assisted living facilities. Hospital-based nursing staffs need to feel comfortable that the hospice clinicians share the same vision and demand the same level of care that staff nurses provide for the end-of-life experience for their patients. Once that relationship bond is created, it is difficult to break. Dottie observes that HOM's clinical people *"are as important as, if not more important than, our marketers."* The clinical people represent the values and mission of HOM. The hospice aides spend the most time caring for patients, and the relationships these aides develop with facility staff create great marketing potential. Nurses look forward to the hospice aides and nurses arriving to care for the very sick patients because it frees them to care for others. Good relationships equal good marketing.

Dottie observed that HOM recently experienced a disruption in its established relationships during an organizational restructuring. Financially and otherwise, the staff reduction was the right thing to do, but it had a short-term negative effect on the important bond between the hospital and nursing home nurses and the hospice registered nurses and social workers. As HOM stabilized, the nursing staff and clinicians established new relationships with new bonds. HOM's quality of service actually improved and its census grew 30 percent year over year between April 2011 and May 2012. HOM is unquestionably the best at what it does, but hospitals and nursing homes can switch very easily to other providers if they desire. The hospital or nursing home administration can just say, "*We want to steer this patient to a different hospice today.*" That represents a big challenge for HOM as it proactively finds it's footing in an increasingly competitive market.

Building Stable Teams: Practice and Reality

HOM has established stable clinical teams and clinical leadership, and that has produced a tremendous amount of energy between the leaders and directors. There is a great team atmosphere at HOM, as evidenced by the significant improvement in staff engagement since the restructuring. Before the restructuring, employee engagement, as measured by the Gallup Q12 instrument, was 3.87:1 engaged staff members to non-engaged employees. Twelve months after the organizational restructuring, the Q12 engagement ratio dramatically improved to 10:1. The clinical leaders have the largest staff and the most influence within the organization. It is critically important that the leaders, directors, and staff establish sound relationships, to keep up with the flow of information and the challenges that need to be resolved. Clinical leaders must remain sharp in their interactions with their staffs to resolve critical day-to-day issues.

Dottie Deremo: *I feel that we are really making progress, yet there are still challenges. We just met yesterday with a really basic challenge. We have a team staff member who is responsible for admissions of new patients and caring for a caseload of current patients. Her clinician inclination is to take care of the patients that we currently have in our program. Then I ask her to bring on another admission, and she will say, "That is great, but I have ten patients who need care now." So, we have good discussions about what care means and how that care is relevant to everyone. Patients need to be cared for, and admissions need to get done. We need staffing models that work for everyone. We are leaner now and can handle a thousand patients a day easily.*

Lack of Respect for Patient and Family Wishes

The Dartmouth Institute for Health Policy and Clinical Practice conducted a study on hospice care for cancer patients. The study demonstrated that end-of-life cancer care varies markedly depending on where patients live and receive care.[6] Even at the top teaching hospitals, the wishes of patients and their families are not always respected. More than one-third of patients dying from cancer spend their last days in an intensive care facility where they continue to receive life support interventions, including chemotherapy and feeding tubes. In fifty academic medical centers, fewer than half the patients received hospice services, with some referrals occurring only within the final few days, when it is too late to make a difference in end-of-life quality.

Despite the progress made in the care of terminally ill patients, a gap exists between the care the dying want and the care they actually receive.[7] Physicians push for more and more treatments even when families protest and demand other options. Physicians often do not have access to all family members who are the decision makers during a healthcare crisis. Healthcare providers often take measures to prolong the life of a dying patient when one family member is ambivalent or requests *"everything possible be done."* In many cases it is the family members who cannot let go; they want to keep the patient in their lives as long as possible or are besieged by guilt.

Counseling Patients on End-of-Life Care

You don't get to choose how you're going to die, or when. You can only decide how you're going to live.

—Joan Baez

Hospice care can be ordered only if a patient is dying, and patients are not always psychologically ready to accept their impending death. When the patient is not ready, then his or her support group is unlikely to be ready, and the physician is also unlikely to be ready. Physicians often indicate that one more treatment will prolong the patient's life. Patients and families who fear death will grasp at any hope, even if the odds are poor at best. Family members often acquiesce to aggressive care without fully understanding the impact on quality of life in the final weeks or months. Some patients with chronic congestive heart failure or end-stage emphysema, for example, may spend two years in the end stage of their disease. These patients cycle in and out of the hospital receiving nothing but episodic care until hospice is ordered.

Physicians and other healthcare professionals who lack thorough training on how to approach the subject of death often fail to counsel patients about their prognosis and the full range of care options, including palliative or hospice care. In the best of circumstances, the patient, the family, and the physician need to have discussions about treatment options at the end of life. This includes the chance of success of an invasive treatment, the patient's overall prognosis, and the patient's expected quality of life with and without treatment. Physicians and healthcare providers need to relearn skills for communicating options for medical care to help patients and their support groups realize their goals for living and for dying.[8]

Ensuring Right of Choice of End-of-Life Care

As corporate director of innovative programs at HOM, Roxanne Roth is responsible for the quality, efficiency, and effectiveness of the care services patients, families, and communities receive. Her responsibilities include promoting a culture of excellence in patient care and ensuring that outcomes related to patient/family/caregiver needs and employee performance and engagement are met.

Roxanne has twenty-five years of nursing experience, which includes a background in oncology, family practice, urgent care, and hospice. She joined HOM in April 1994 and has worked on several research projects, including the Robert Wood Johnson–funded Palliative Care Program. She used this experience to design and develop the @HOMe Support™ Program, which was initiated under her guidance in the fall of 2006. Since then, she has continued to oversee this innovative advanced illness service to provide care to all of her patients.

Many patients prefer to die in the comfort of their home, surrounded by the family, friends, and possessions that gave meaning to their life. In studies of patients with advanced chronic illness, 43–50 percent preferred to receive care at home even when their recovery appeared hopeless.[9] Hospice care makes that preference possible by offering pain and symptom management as well as psychological and spiritual support. An interdisciplinary team of physicians, nurses, social workers, aides, dietitians, therapists, chaplains, counselors, and volunteers, all with end-of-life expertise, provides patient care. HOM excels at helping patients and their families plan for their last days. The staff sits with patients, talks to them, cries with them, helps them consider what they want for their funeral, what music they want, what gifts they want given, and, most important, how they want to be remembered. The staff also works directly with families to plan how they want their loved one remembered.

Several studies have shown that patients who talk with their families or physicians about their preferences for end-of-life care have less anxiety and feel more control over their medical care and their disease. They feel their physician truly understands their needs, and they feel more comfortable about their decision-making. When the patient becomes too ill to participate or is unable to make his or her wishes known, the family and the physician make decisions based on what they "think" the patient wants.[10] Often, families make guesses because they really do not know what the loved one wants and have not had the opportunity to discuss the issues with him or her.

HOM's interdisciplinary teams provide invaluable support to patients and their families. Often a nurse or social worker will sit down with the patient or with one or more family members to talk about what to expect during the dying process and to paint a picture of what will gradually happen as death approaches. Even with that knowledge, death can be brutal and the suffering unbearable.[11] There are limits to what can be achieved, even with superb interdisciplinary end-of-life medical care. Transparency is critical: patients have a right to know what will take place and how their bodies will begin to shut down. Families need to know that death is natural and can take place without the implementation of extreme measures in the final few days.

Providing care options is critical because the choice is the patient's, in conjunction with family, friends, and other support group members. The choices should not be all or nothing. Whether care is to be provided at the very end of life or during the final twenty-four months, the patient and the family must make the care choices that will provide the outcome they desire. "*Living well*" has different meanings for different patients. Patients and their support groups must understand the available choices and be able to meaningfully discuss care options with their physicians. Caring for a dying patient can be an extraordinary opportunity for personal growth for family, friends, and support group members. Surrounded by family and friends, the patient can face his or her own death comfortably and with dignity.

Well-supported families translate to well-supported patients. Families need to be empowered so that they can make the right decisions about end-of-life care for their loved one. As family members observe the impending death of their loved one, they must deal with their own fear of death and with questions about the meaning of life. Death means that a loved one will be taken away—forever. Consequently, families want to be asked about their goals and wishes for what will happen after their loved one is gone. Death is a natural part of life, coming in waves of pain and suffering. But ever so gradually, the pain of death recedes, and living begins again for the survivors.

The secret of a good old age is simply an honorable pact with solitude.

—Gabriel Garcia Marquez

One Patient's Story: Life at Home after the Hospital

Roxanne Roth: *There was one elderly woman, an 86 year old, who was being cared for by her son (who was also ill). When HOM received the referral, the patient had had multiple hospitalizations, including one stay at a nursing home. Her hospitalizations were for many comorbid conditions including stroke, skin breakdowns, difficulty swallowing, infections related to pressure ulcers, a urinary tract infection, a heart condition, renal insufficiencies, and early dementia. All of these conditions were chronic and not going away.*

While she was in the hospital, she had had a lot of behavioral issues and major outbursts; she simply did not want to be there. When HOM arrived, she had another outburst, but her son told us that it was fairly mild compared with what had happened in the hospital. She had a visiting physician who encouraged her son to take her back to the hospital, but she absolutely refused. So often it is the physician who is afraid to talk about death—they can't give up trying every last measure to keep the patient alive.

At home, in familiar surroundings, the woman slowly began to feel better. Within the first benefit period, the pressure ulcers were relieved, and she was able to take a long-term indwelling catheter out. She was able to feed herself and began to show improvement in health and mood. During the review period, we noticed that she was taking twelve different medications, which she hated. Each medication was prescribed for a specific reason, but they were counteracting each other and were partially responsible for her outbursts. This elderly woman together with her son decided to discontinue all the medications except for one aspirin and a stool softener. She improved further.

The critical piece in hospice care is providing for the psychosocial needs of both the patient and her family. This can be hard for nurses, who are trained to pay attention only to the patient. This elderly woman's care team gained their patient's trust by finding out what was important to her, including small things such as making her favorite coffee and bringing it to her. The nurse took pains to create a relationship with her patient, getting to know what made her happy and making an extra effort to deliver what she needed.

Often when you pay attention to a family member, the patient will do better. Attention giving can be as simple as doing the dishes or sitting with the patient so that the caregiver can take a break. Teaching caregivers different ways to care for the patient makes it easier on them and on their loved one.

Acute changes can come on suddenly. Caregivers need to know what to look for. For example, we taught the elderly woman's son to watch for his mother's shifting in her chair [as a sign of discomfort] *because she couldn't articulate what was making her uncomfortable. The son needed to be able to call someone at two o'clock in the morning for help in determining whether whatever was happening was an emergency—and if it was an emergency, what were the different options for care, especially because his mother so desperately wanted to stay out of the hospital. He needed to know what resources were available to him so that he could take care of his mother's needs and keep her at home.*

Focusing on Caregiver Support

HOM has created support programs with a focus on the caregiver. Many times it is the caregiver who calls at 3 a.m. to have the patient admitted to the hospital because the family member is thoroughly exhausted and needs a break. But with every visit to the emergency room and with every hospital admission, costs rise, and the final bill for the hospital stay could well exceed $40,000. Then the patient goes into long-term care for 120 days of rehabilitation, and finally the patient receives home care. When the limit for covered home visits is reached, then everything stops. Patients with advancing chronic illness can go through six to ten of these cycles over the eighteen months of care. Then the cycle begins again, a cycle that misuses medical resources and likely ends in death.

"*Caregivers*" are generally unpaid relatives or friends called upon to assist patients who have a chronic illness or disease. As patients grow older, the role of the caregiver becomes that much more important, both functionally and economically. Caregivers talk to physicians or nurses about medications, help bathe and/or dress frail patients, and assist them with their daily activities. The role of the caregiver is critical, but caregivers need to look after themselves as well. Taking daily walks, resting, getting enough sleep, seeing a movie, shopping, and being with nature—all these activities help revive caregivers and enable them to take better care of their loved one.[12]

Fostering Spiritual and Cultural Connections

Just as a candle cannot burn without fire, men cannot live without a spiritual life.

Education, clinical information, psychological support, and self-management offer patients the means for dealing with pain, making good health decisions, coping with crises, and handling end-of-life care. Attention to detail is critically important when it comes to dealing with frail patients. Further, caregiver support and patient support interweave, with each reinforcing the other. Caring behaviors do make a difference. The more HOM focuses on the individual patient and the more the staff creates a caring and healing environment, the better the outcomes for the patient and his or her family.[13] Researchers have found that when nurses take over the care of terminally ill patients, satisfaction scores go up. A better-supported family means a better-supported patient.

Spirituality—both patients' and staffs'—is important to overall hospice care. The more the healthcare staff focuses on their own spiritual consciousness, the more the staff can support the patient in his or her spiritual quest. Madeline Leininger's book, *Cultural Care Diversity and Universality*,[14] addresses care for patients from different cultures. She fervently believes that people from other cultures who come to the United States deserve respectful care delivered by sensitive professionals fully cognizant of their unique needs. Leininger believes there are several "universal" actions that 40 percent of patients representing eighty cultures want for their own care. These actions are identified below.

Leininger's Five Assumptions on Caring
1. Care is essential for human growth and survival, and to face death.

2. There can be no curing without caring.

3. Expressions of human care vary among all the cultures in the world.

4. Therapeutic nursing care can only occur when cultural care values, expressions, or practices are known and used explicitly.

5. Nursing is a transcultural care profession and discipline.
(Leininger, 1994)

Culture molds society through its unwritten rules and guides behaviors from cradle to grave. Cultural beliefs and traditions define family life; dictate roles and responsibilities; and determine decision-making, resource distribution, and problem-solving methods. Culture influences how families cope with stress and whether they will seek help from outsiders. HOM's staff has learned not to judge patients from other cultures through the lens of their own culture. They have learned that patients' individual needs, history, and cultural experiences determine their ability to tell the staff what they want for their care. "Knowing thyself" before knowing and judging others is critical in working with patients and families from other cultures.

When the nurse queries the patient about his or her culture, she is searching for guidance on how to interact with other members of diverse ethnic and cultural communities. The answers she seeks help her to understand the expectations and dynamics within families and determine what kind of religious (or nonreligious) service will be most acceptable. They help the clinicians identify trusted persons who can be called upon for help. Finally, they provide insight into promising approaches for spreading the word about available amenities, including bringing spiritual leaders in to pray with patients, food preparation, laundry services, house cleaners, and dog walkers. All of these services reduce the pressure on family members so that they can concentrate on their dying loved one.

How Life Goals Affect Patient Attitudes about Death

Self-determination theory (SDT) postulates that the type of goals people aspire to remains critically important for well-being and integrity as they age, face chronic illness, and consider the end of life.[15] Older adults who have attained intrinsic (internal) goals such as community service, personal growth, and development of meaningful relationships express psychological needs for autonomy, competence, and relatedness. Older adults who report having set and achieved more intrinsic goals during their life are more accepting of their own death and much more "ready to die." As older adults age, they are more likely to draw upon past personal experiences and integrate those experiences with their final destiny. The attainment of intrinsic goals is conducive to aging individuals' psychological well-being, and to their ultimate acceptance of death. Erik Erikson (1980) notes that in the later stages of life, there is a *"meaningful interplay between beginning and end as well as some finite sense of summary and possibly, a more active anticipation of dying."*

In contrast, older adults who have been concerned primarily with extrinsic (external) goals such as financial success, power, beauty, and social recognition want to validate their ego by making good impressions on others. Older people who highly value their physical appearance are more likely to be repulsed at the deterioration in their good looks, and to feel bad about how they appear to others. Power, with all of its false promises, has a similar hold on older adults who give it great value; they often wince when a younger person takes their place at the top. The quest for financial success, measured in big paychecks and fat investment accounts, has very much the same lure. Older adults who continuously need to attain new extrinsic goals of fortune, beauty, power, or recognition find it hard to alleviate death anxiety and stress.

Wealth doesn't change who you are, it only reveals you to yourself.
—Dayo Oloma

Medicare Managed-Care versus Fee-for-Service Outcomes

Dottie explains the day-to-day variations in HOM's census figures by describing the effect of weekends on census calculations.

> Dottie Deremo: *Monday census figures are critical to HOM's bottom line. Deaths and admissions occur over the weekend, and it takes time to collect and reconcile census figures to produce an accurate Monday census report. HOM's census numbers often dip on Monday and Tuesday, only to rise again on Wednesday. Tuesday is usually the lowest census day, and Friday is usually the highest census day of the week. On a linear regression, HOM wants to match Monday-to-Monday and Tuesday-to-Tuesday metrics. That allows apples-to-apples comparisons from week to week. HOM*

figures are constantly changing with admissions and deaths, so generating accurate figures requires well-defined data processes and systems.

For individuals in hospice care, Medicare pays for 80 percent of their expenses at a maximum of $146 per day. The payment covers all services, medications, and durable medical equipment (DME). Expenses during the last days of care are often huge, although the money stream remains the same. A study, which was conducted by Ellen McCarthy, compared hospice use among Medicare managed-care and fee-for-service (FFS) patients dying with cancer.[16] The study found that Medicare patients with managed-care insurance had consistently higher rates of hospice use and significantly longer hospice stays (two months or more) than did those with FFS insurance (less than two weeks). Patients with managed-care insurance have much better opportunities to benefit from hospice care than do patients with FFS insurance. When patients are admitted to hospice so late, families do not have sufficient time to care for them or to benefit from hospice care.

The transition from chronic illness to death is challenging both for patients and for families—and it is very expensive. In the United States, patients in the last year of life consume 10–12 percent of all healthcare spending and 27 percent of the total Medicare budget. In addition, up to 30 percent of Medicare spending for patients during their last two years of life is unnecessary and does little to improve their health.[17] But letting go is difficult for patients and their families. Physicians, too, have a difficult time letting go and will often hold out for more treatments, more chemotherapy, or another surgery. It is important to address these systemic pressures because the more the health system can reduce frantic end-of-life surgeries, chemotherapy treatments, medications, and use of intensive care units, the more hospice and palliative care can ease the minds of patients and their families.

Dottie Deremo: *The very ill need a lot of support in the home.* [People] *can have two to ten crises in the final twenty-four months of life. Signing on patients for the* [DMC Michigan Pioneer ACO] *Personalized Care at Home Program may take up to nine months because hospice looks at two to three hundred patients at a time to determine if they are at end-stage illness. Hospice of Michigan research indicates that its special program for end-stage-illness patients saves 30-plus percent in medical costs while providing higher quality care and reducing stress for caregivers during patients' last twenty-four months of life.*

Hospice Marketing: It's All in the Name

The logistics of providing hospice care for Rogers City, located in a very rural part of Michigan, and for the heart of urban Detroit are difficult. The same standard of care needs to be applied in these very different communities. There are only a limited number of facilities in Michigan's rural areas, but Southeast Michigan has a variety of facility levels: among them, hospitals, home health care, and long-term care facilities. In areas such as Alpena, Michigan, HOM has 70 percent of the market, but in metropolitan Detroit, HOM has at least sixty competitors. The for-profit companies do not compete in rural areas like Alpena in northern Michigan.

Instead, for-profits companies focus their efforts on the densest markets. Since metropolitan Detroit is now saturated with hospice programs, the for-profits are moving into the next tier of populated areas, like Grand Rapids in west Michigan. A large out-of-state for-profit company that competes with HOM has as many marketers in the city of Detroit as HOM has for the remainder of the state of Michigan. Therefore, HOM's market share in Detroit is less than 20 percent. To make things more difficult, HOM's sixty Detroit competitors ride under HOM's "white hat"—most patients who are receiving hospice care believe they are receiving it from HOM.

HOM is working to rebrand itself—to differentiate itself from all its competitors. Seymour M. "Skip" Roberts, a HOM Board member with a deep understanding of marketing, is donating his time to the rebranding effort. From the old school of marketing, Skip demands excellence. He is pushing HOM and pushing its public relations firms to define what excellence means. Most hospice organizations emphasize the "touchy-feely" aspects of care, with messages such as, "Hospice offers hope to patients and families." HOM's advertising reinforces the proposition that hospice is wonderful, *but it does not differentiate Hospice of Michigan from other hospice organizations.* HOM has decided that it needs to take a stand and discuss what makes it unique and critically important in this competitive market. To that end, HOM's vision is to innovate end-of-life care and to role model the way for America. As part of its rebranding effort as the expert in end-of-life care in Michigan, HOM is now advertising on television in all its key markets highlighting a HOM clinical expert from each hospice and palliative care discipline of medicine, nursing, social work, spiritual care, hospice aide, grief support, and volunteers.

The Development of a Leader

Dottie Deremo started her career in 1969 as a diploma graduate from a hospital school of nursing because it was affordable. Her first job was in critical care, an emerging field for nursing. Dottie loved the challenge and relative independence in critical care that allowed her to apply her clinical judgment in difficult clinical situations.

Within two years, Dottie was back in school at Wayne State University (WSU) College of Nursing in their BSN completion program. Dottie recognized she had to acquire more knowledge to become a better nurse. At WSU, she learned about the emerging role of master's degreed clinical nurse specialists prepared to be nurse practitioners in primary care (CNS/NP). Independent nursing practice was very appealing to Dottie's entrepreneurial spirit and unending thirst for knowledge. Dottie plowed straight through her

BSN and MSN programs becoming one of the first master's degree prepared NPs in the state. Immediately upon completion of her graduate degree, she accepted a joint faculty/practice position at Michigan State University (MSU).

The position at MSU allowed Dottie to teach nurses and medical students in both the graduate nursing and osteopathic medical programs about collaborative practice. She was also responsible for setting up a primary care collaborative practice clinic with the medical faculty as learning laboratory where both the nursing and medical students could witness good patient care.

Within one year, Dottie was recruited back to WSU to teach graduate nursing students in the CNS/NP program. Unfortunately, the only clinical placements available to the students were physician practices in which the majority did not have CNS/NP role models. Dottie and two other CNS/NP faculty lamented about this lack of CNS/NP role-models. This deficit instilled a medical model of primary care in their students and de-emphasized the expanded role of advanced practice nursing. To address this problem, the three of them came to the conclusion that they needed to develop a nursing group practice so that their graduate students would have a real-life, advanced practice nursing learning laboratory to learn to become "maxi-nurses" rather than "mini-physicians" with a little bit of nursing thrown in.

For Dottie Deremo, creating the nursing group practice from scratch at the Detroit Medical Center (DMC) in 1977 was a wonderful experience. She was able to take what she had learned as a nurse practitioner, investigate organizational shortcomings, and integrate them both into a holistic approach focused on leadership and outcomes. When Dottie and her two faculty nurse practitioner colleagues first arrived at the DMC, they started their clinic with two examining rooms, a file cabinet, and a phone. From this modest beginning, these three nurse practitioners built a practice from scratch and within two years had 2,800 clients.

Dottie could do a complete history and physical and not leave a patch of skin unexamined, but it took her three hours to complete one exam. That patient received a quality exam, but there were twenty patients waiting for their turn, and for them it was not quality. What patients needed was timely care delivered with quality and with compassion. No one else was to blame for the lack of a caring exam, not the nursing nor the hospital administration. But Dottie learned a lot about taking full responsibility for running a good practice and delivering excellent leadership.

Dottie recalls her mother telling her repeatedly, *"Don't complain about something if you are not going to do something about it."*

Dottie found herself asking, *"What if I could take some of these crazy ideas and inoculate them into rigid health systems? What if I could mix the military and the monastery?"* She wanted to see both good work and excellent healing in a sacred space within a holistic organization.

Dottie observes that there are two types of managers: a *"head and hands"* group and a *"heart and soul"* group. In the head and hands crowd, the "head" creates the strategy and the tactics, the analytics and the principles to organize and plan the future. The "hands" managers are all about the doing, the execution, and the drive for results. The "heart" managers are all about people, taking care of and engaging them. This group tugs at the emotions. The "soul" crowd creates a vision that moves people to do something for the greater good.

Some leaders can be described as 25 percent leaders, meaning that they are all about execution (hands) or all about plans and strategies (head). Then there are the 50 percent leaders: the head and hands group or the heart and soul group, but the rest of the organizational potential is left on the table. Real leadership is holistic, integrating the soul, the heart, the head, and the hands. Real leaders maximize both organizational and human potential by giving and engaging 100 percent of themselves and their staff. These leaders achieve the right outcomes for HOM patients and their families and for the community.

It was in 1992, while working full time as chief nursing officer for Henry Ford Health System (HFHS) and raising her children, that

Dottie went back to school for her master's in health administration and policy. She was expecting to be promoted to a CEO position within HFHS—until a search firm contacted her requesting that she be a candidate for CEO of HOM. By the time the firm contacted her again, eight weeks later, her mother had died in hospice care. She agreed to do one interview—and the rest is history. Dottie knew that HOM was the place she wanted to work. It was a small enough space to test her theories and determine if they could work.

> Dottie Deremo: *I became a CEO because no one has the same feeling about insurance that they do about hospice. Last week, I used my office phone to call an office administrator about a minor medical procedure. The woman who answered the phone saw the "Hospice of Michigan" ID on her phone. She has incredible regard for HOM because of this halo around us. At the end of the call, she said, "God bless you for what you do." That is why I came here. It is nice to be associated with a company that has a mission like this one's.*

For patients, end of life is a time to say goodbye and to complete unfinished business. For families, it is a time to say, *"I love you,"* *"Please forgive me,"* *"Thank you for all you have done for me,"* and *"I forgive you."*[18] When these things are taken care of before someone dies, the survivors move into the future sad, but also hopeful. That is a far cry from the situation for families whose loved one is trapped in a hospital bed attached to machines with tubes and wires. Such a situation makes it very difficult for families to provide the kind of loving support they want to offer at the end of life.

Careers often unfold and map themselves when we do not force them but instead remain open and educate ourselves. Education opens the mind and helps us develop critical thinking skills. Dottie observes that the lessons she learned as a nurse practitioner have helped her more in her job as HOM's CEO than did what she learned in her master's program in health administration and policy. As a nurse practitioner, she learned to use her interpersonal skills, to speak and write convincingly, and to understand the dynamics of personalities in groups. Softer skills like those are as important to a leader as are the harder skills of using analytical tools or understanding a balance sheet.[19] As Dottie's mother told her, *"Honey, you can have it all. You just can't have it all at once."*

One Nurse Leader's Accomplishments

- In her leadership role, Dottie has grown hospice care so that it now serves more than 1,100 patients a day across fifty-six Michigan counties.

- Dottie, in partnership with Steven Grant, M.D., recently signed a contract to help manage the sickest patients in the Detroit Medical Center's new accountable care organization, thus saving 30-plus percent in medical costs over 24 months.

- She has stabilized the relationships between the nursing staff and clinicians, and as a result HOM's quality of service actually improved and its census grew 30 percent year over year between April 2011 and May 2012.

- She restructured the staff, and as a result employee engagement, as measured by the Gallup Q12 instrument, was 3.87:1 engaged staff members to non-engaged employees. Twelve months after the organizational restructuring, the Q12 engagement ratio dramatically improved to 10:1.

- She has improved the spiritual connections between her staff and all of her patients. They have learned that patients' individual needs, history, and cultural experiences determine their ability to tell the staff what they want for their care.

- She has worked closely with Mr. Roberts, a HOM board

member, to discuss what makes HOM unique and critically important in this competitive market.

- She has taught her special brand of real leadership. Real leaders maximize both organizational and human potential by giving 100 percent of their time and unique talents to achieving the right outcomes for HOM patients and their families and for the community.

- Roxanne also provides her innovative approach to care through the @HOMe Support™ Program, which since its fall 2006 inception, has grown to cover end-of life care in hospitals, nursing homes, and family homes. Roxanne reaches across all departments to promote a culture-of-excellence program in patient care and to ensure that the desired patient/family/caregiver outcomes are met.

Conclusion

With HOM's national reputation, Dottie believes that through her work, she can change end-of-life care for America and offer a cocoon of support for patients, their families, and their support groups. As one of the largest hospice organizations in the country, HOM has specialists in many areas, including pediatric hospice, pain management, research, care for people with advanced dementia and AIDS. Among its 600 employees, it counts more board-certified hospice physicians and nurses than at other hospices.[20] HOM understood that physicians were the key to improving end-of-life care and began offering educational programs to physicians and healthcare providers through its education and research center, the Maggie Allesee Center for Quality of Life. Dr. Diane Meier, national director of the Center to Advance Palliative Care, has called Hospice of Michigan the "Harvard of hospice in American."

Dottie Deremo: *At Hospice of Michigan, we know from thirty years of experience with thousands of individuals and their families that physicians are trusted advisors, and that patients want to be the decision makers as long as possible. We created programs for physicians to enhance education on end-of-life care and tools to empower patients and families. We believe that quality care at the end of life is essential and that patients deserve the best our medical systems can offer.*

Actions for Nurse Practitioners

Question for Reflection

How are you creating an environment in which everyone is encouraged to stretch beyond what they think is possible? What are you doing to create energy, excitement, and a sense of personal investment in patients, families, physicians, and staff? How are you exhibiting great leadership using a holistic approach?

Showing Appreciation

- Reinforce the concept that everyone's work is important.
- Show appreciation for the simple things that nurses do for patients and their families.

Example:

Bedside nurses want to be appreciated for all they do to help patients. For example, the nurse described earlier gained the patient's trust by making coffee at home and bringing it to her. She created a relationship with her patient by sitting next to her, holding her hand, and encouraging her to talk. She took over the dishwashing so that the patient's caregiver son could have some free time.

Encouraging Involvement

- Create a positive environment that encourages acceptance of others' ideas.
- Convey a sense of humor, and encourage fun in the workplace.

Example:

Bedside nurses rarely have the opportunity to get together around a great idea and genuinely influence a project. Go out of your way to include as many staff as possible in planning. Getting everyone's opinion can help to ensure that everyone feels ownership over your project. Make meetings fun. People want to come to meetings where there is laugher, even if the project is serious.

Facing Spirituality and Cultural Peace

- Patients need to find their own cultural destiny and assistance in searching for their own spiritual peace.
- Nurses need guidance on how to interact with patients from different cultures and different family dynamics.

Example:

Nurses need to find out about the patient and their individual culture and their own beliefs about what he or she believes. They also need to query the patient about available amenities such as spiritual leaders to pray, food preparation, and laundry services. Try to understand what the patient wants, their history and cultural experiences. Search for ways really know the patient through their own eyes.

Challenging the Nursing Staff

- Identify criteria that will help nurses (and family members) recognize the early signs of "danger" in the patient.
- Reinforce the concept that mistakes are learning opportunities, not opportunities for placing blame.

Example:

Help others reduce their fear of risk taking and failure by eliminating blame and finger pointing. While still holding staff accountable for their actions, make it clear that it is only through mistakes that learning takes place. Maintain a nonpunitive atmosphere. When it is critical to getting your point across, demonstrate emotion—even frustration—with staff.

Becoming a Great Leader

- Real leadership springs from a holistic approach, combining the heart, the soul, the head, and the hands.
- Great leaders capture 100 percent of the organization and its people's potential.

Example:

Managers fall into two camps: (1) with their heads, they create strategy, organize and plan; with their hands they execute the plan. Or (2) they move people to a higher purpose and engage people from their emotions. What can you do to achieve the outcomes that patients, families, and communities deserve?

CHAPTER FOUR

Nurse Practitioners Empowering Rural Women: Cancer Screening for the Underserved

The Impact of Breast and Cervical Cancer

In 2007, the American Cancer Society estimated that in the United States, 178,480 women would be diagnosed with invasive breast cancer and 40,460 women would die from the disease. During that same period, 11,150 U.S. women would be diagnosed with invasive cervical cancer and 3,670 would die. The West Virginia Cancer Registry noted that from 1999 to 2003, breast cancer was the most commonly diagnosed cancer among West Virginia women and the leading cause of cancer-related deaths in women aged 25–44. During that same period, cervical cancer was the tenth most commonly diagnosed cancer among West Virginia women (third among women aged 25–44 years) and the third leading cause of cancer-related deaths among women in that age group.[1] Cancer incidences are elevated in rural Appalachia, suggesting lack of access to good cancer healthcare.

Many rural women are confused about breast and cervical cancer screening programs, especially the fact that these programs may be publicly supported. Unfortunately, these women often receive inaccurate or dated information about cancer prevention, screening, and treatments. If rural women are to get the care they rightfully deserve, they need access to accurate, up-to-date information.

Stepping Up to the Plate

Twice a year, Dr. Wendy Grube takes nurse practitioner and midwifery students in the University of Pennsylvania's "Well Women Health Care" to Webster Springs, West Virginia, to the Webster County Memorial Hospital to conduct breast and cervical cancer screenings for women in the surrounding mountain regions. Wendy's goals are to provide vital screening services and to tap local communication channels to disseminate accurate cancer information while counteracting local women's skepticism about the quality of the healthcare available to them and their lack of trust in providers.[2]

In 2006, when Wendy saw a request through Appalnet, the Appalachian professionals' listserve, for help for a health fair in Webster Springs, she responded. At the invitation of Mountains of Hope member Jean Tenney, Wendy and five of her students traveled to Webster Springs, population 800, to participate in the October fair. Then in February 2007, the Webster County Cancer Education Project conducted its first women's community workshops on colorectal, breast, and cervical cancer. The Mountains of Hope project comprises twenty collaborative partners: local individuals, churches, community organizations, and regional groups.[3] The project began when Mrs. Tenney went to a storytelling workshop with Mountains of Hope; she wanted to tell stories about cancer and address the need to care for and support each other throughout the course of the disease.

The West Virginia Breast and Cervical Cancer Screening Program (WVBCCSP) is a comprehensive public health program that helps uninsured or underinsured women gain access to breast and cervical cancer screening services. Screening and early detection of cancer reduces death rates and improves treatment options. A combination of federal monies, West Virginia state funds, and Medicaid benefits funds the program. Since the program's inception in 1991, the WVBCCSP has enrolled more than 107,000 women and provided more than 209,000 Pap tests, 136,000 mammograms, and 198,000 breast exams.[4]

Following the WVBCCSP workshops, several local women participated in a focus group about cervical cancer. Their comments revealed misunderstandings about the risks of that cancer. Information women receive from family and neighbors is often inadequate. In addition, many of the women attending the workshops could not afford a Pap test or a breast mammogram. The WVBCCSP then decided to offer a free screening clinic for eligible Webster County women.

Because Wendy and her students had participated in the health fair and because of their interest in the Webster Springs community, WVBCCSP invited them to return to Webster Springs to conduct breast and pelvic exams and Pap tests at the Webster County Memorial Hospital and Webster County Health Department.[5] Since 2006, Wendy and her students have returned twelve times to partner with rural West Virginia women and collaborate in addressing their unique healthcare needs.

Wendy Grube: *It was critical for me to become involved with their community to better understand the sociocultural influences affecting reproductive healthcare and screening practices. It turned out to be incredibly rewarding, and these wonderful women have become my infinitely patient teachers.*

Webster County: A Profile

While Webster Springs, West Virginia, does advertise tobacco cessation and obesity classes through the cancer screening sessions and primary care physicians care for patients with chronic diseases, the county still lags behind other counties in providing preventive care for heart disease, chronic obstructive pulmonary disease (COPD), and hypertension. Smokeless tobacco, alcohol, and substance abuse are prevalent.

In Webster County, West Virginia, some residents lack health insurance and experience elevated rates of poverty and unemployment.[6] As in the rest of the United States, the ranks of West Virginia's uninsured continue to grow. A Gallup poll found that 17.1 percent of U.S. adults did not have health insurance in 2011, a significant increase from the 16.4 percent uninsured in 2010. Unemployment and underemployment contribute to this trend, as does the rising cost of healthcare.[7]

The Webster County Memorial Hospital provides basic screenings such as Pap tests and breast exams, but those needing cancer treatment must leave the area. The nearest cancer facilities are from two hours to a day's ride away on winding mountain roads to cities like Clarksburg, Summersville, or Charleston, West Virginia. People often team up to share the cost of the drive and get their cancer treatments in hospitals that can administer chemotherapy and radiation and can perform the necessary surgeries. Nevertheless, travel costs to maintain a treatment regimen are often prohibitively high.

Convincing Rural Women to Be Screened

The WVBCCSP does a lot of advertising on the radio, in newspapers, and on television. Church and local volunteers send notices to people who have attended previous screenings and walk door to door and talk to women in the community who have not yet been screened. It is a tight community, and often when a neighbor comes knocking, the resident will agree to go for a screening if the neighbor goes as well. What really motivates women to be screened is personal stories from neighbor volunteers about their own experiences with breast or cervical cancer. Women in communities where it is not the norm to go to a hospital for a screening will likely not go.

On March 15, 2011, at a local church not far from the hotel where Wendy Grube, her students, and Sydney Lentz were staying, a group of church volunteers led by Mrs. Jean Tenney were putting on a play titled "Mountains of Hope." Mrs. Tenney had attended a storytelling workshop where she learned how to transport personal experiences with cancer into the oral tradition. Volunteers wrote the script for the play, which featured people telling their stories of how they had faced cancer and learned to feel the fear, deal with the truth, and get to the other side of the cancer. Personal stories such as these can be moving, funny, and very transformational. Participants spoke from their hearts about their experiences learning to cope with cancer and translating pain into insight.

At the end of the play, members of the audience stood up and spoke about friends and family who had died, who fought cancer and survived, and who continue to fight the disease. A student of Wendy's spoke about her parents, who died within months of each other. Through her tears, she recounted her memories of them and explained how cancer had robbed her of their love and support. These testimonies bring home what cancer means and make those who hear them think differently about how screenings can save lives.

The Face of Webster County Healthcare

Webster County Memorial Hospital has one and a half doctors—Dr. Luke McElwain and his wife, Dr. Melanie Pavone (a part-time physician)—and a physician assistant (PA), Debra Cutlip. When women come to the hospital, they usually do not see the doctor; instead they see the PA. Debbie has received training beyond that needed for PA certification and takes on challenges beyond what her credentials represent. She is an excellent clinician and works hard at what she does, but she is limited. Dr. McElwain provides consultation and treats patients with multiple co-morbid illnesses, many of whom require care that goes beyond his training. However, McElwain is the only doctor available to these patients. The nearest gynecologist is more than two hours away over winding mountain roads, and the nearest specialists who can treat patients with co-morbid illnesses are in towns even further away.

Rhonda Hayhurst, a registered nurse (RN) who works for the WVBCCSP, is another local source for women needing healthcare services. As can other RNs who have passed a competency test,

Rhonda can do breast and cervical cancer screenings and enter the results into the system. RNs are stepping up to do mammograms and Pap tests in rural areas lacking physicians, NPs, midwives, and PAs, but they cannot diagnose and treat what they may uncover. Even when rural women have access to an NP or a PA, there are limits to their practice. Few trained NPs choose rural areas, and many leave after only a few years, for better compensation, better lifestyle choices, and higher caliber healthcare facilities.

Kathy Chapman, the CEO of Webster County Memorial Hospital, has access to an indigents' fund, as does every hospital in every state. To limit potential abuse of these funds, however, applicants must work their way through layers of bureaucracy. To qualify for the fund, individuals must submit all their medical bills, disclose their income, provide their Social Security number, present their birth certificate, and write an essay explaining why they need the funds. The question Kathy Chapman asks is this: *"How can I make this funding available to the people who really need it? Can you imagine someone who is severely ill trying to jump through all these hoops?"*

Here are just a few examples of rural women who cannot afford the treatment they need: One woman with both chronic obstructive pulmonary disease and bronchitis was breathing hard and inhaling 2–2.5 liters of air almost continuously. She had signed the "against medical advice" (AMA) form over and over because there were no funds for her care. A chest x-ray costs $125, plus another $200 for a radiologist to read it. Another woman had paid off all but $1,000 of her bill for an earlier hysterectomy. Now she has severe pelvic pain but will not go to the hospital because of her former bills. Rural women without health insurance are very afraid of racking up bills. Women often refuse to acknowledge their pain and suffering even when they know they should see a physician.

Distrust of the Medical Community

Is nonparticipation in healthcare services a result of dissonance between the culture of a given population and the culture of medicine?

Appalachian Culture

- Self-sufficiency
- Importance of kinship
- Ties to the land
- Rejection of mainstream ideas of status
- Conservative Christian view
- Dedication to tradition
- Distrust in and avoidance of conventional healthcare
- Self-care, folk remedies

Culture of Medicine

- Unconditional belief in science
- Standard definitions of health and illness
- Emphasis on specific preventive care practices
- Unique language
- Values compliance
- Professional deference and hierarchical structure
- Rituals of examination

Provided by Dr. Wendy Grube, Director of the Women's Health Care Nurse Practitioner Program at the University of Pennsylvania

Some women have undergone procedures with no understanding of why those procedures were performed. For example, after one woman gave birth to her last son, the physician performed a loop electrosurgical excision procedure (LEEP). LEEP uses a thin wire loop electrode attached to an electrosurgical generator. The generator transmits a painless electric current that cuts away the affected cervical tissue around the loop.[8] The woman did not understand why the physician did what he did and was afraid to ask him to explain. Women deserve to know what is happening to them and why. Denied basic information, many women have good reason to fear medicine.

One woman repeated this statement from a physician: *"Don't worry your pretty little head about such things. You don't need to worry about what body parts you have. I am just going to take care of it."* The woman was embarrassed to ask what body parts she had or should have. She was made to feel that she didn't even know something as basic as that.

How Religious Beliefs Influence Medical Care

Religious beliefs represent an important factor within the Appalachian community. Women of all ages may not seek care because it is God's will if they get cancer. Religious beliefs provide order in an otherwise unpredictable world.[9] That said, many Appalachians address both their faith and the potential benefits of seeking medical care when they are diagnosed with cancer. Health professionals can provide direction on cancer cures; however, they must understand the balance between an individual's faith and effective cancer control. Only through this balance can health professionals provide to their patients the comfort they seek.

Too-High Cancer Death Rates in Appalachia

Hope is living with courage and confidence, not fear.
—Penny Boldrey

Women living in Appalachia are vulnerable to dying of cervical and breast cancer because many avoid the screening programs that could identify these diseases in the early stages, when treatment can be effective. Despite government subsidies to educate and enroll women in screening programs throughout high-risk areas, the rate at which women are screened is inadequate.[10] Focus groups and surveys reveal that rural women gain most of their information about cancer from family, neighbors, and friends rather than from health professionals. The goal for all of Appalachia is to improve knowledge about cancer.

Increasing cancer education involves using local communication channels to broadcast accurate cancer information while at the same time reinforcing physicians and health systems as important sources of accurate, up-to-date information.[11]

From 1994 through 1998, the age-adjusted cancer mortality rate for all of Appalachia (173.1 per 100,000 people) was a statistically significant 4 percent greater than the rate for the United States as a whole (166.7). Rural counties in Appalachia experienced an even higher cancer mortality rate (176.1). For all cancers, the rate among Appalachian males (225.5 per 100,000) is significantly higher than the rate for females (140.5 per 100,000).[12]

No woman should die from cervical cancer; it is 99.9 percent preventable. Women need to be introduced to screening early, and then kept in the screening loop. People need to be informed about treatments for various cancers, but the more important step is education about the value of prevention and screening in saving lives. All women need to be screened for breast, cervical, and colorectal cancer. The alternative—not being screened—is not humane. Women need to stand up for their rights to affordable healthcare. The one and only purpose Wendy Grube and her nursing students serve during their trips to West Virginia is cancer screening. If a screening reveals one or more primary care issues, Grube and her students must refer the woman to other sources of care in other facilities.

Wendy Grube: *We are not of this community and need to trust that there are other resources for primary care. We have one job and that is to do the screening. We are here to do Pap tests and that is all. We may not see the results of that Pap smear or know if the woman gets proper care based on the results. We need to trust that good healthcare will be provided and these women will be properly treated. Maybe later in life, we can come back and take care of these women, but not now.*

The Dangers of "Hit-and-Run" Care

A case study: *Twenty years ago, a woman had a car accident in which a brake went through her knee. Since then, she has been having recurrent falls. [After the latest incident,] she had a fractured patella and probably cellulitis. The NPs and midwifery students brought in Wendy because the knee was swollen and hot. They wheeled the woman down to the emergency room to have the swelling removed and the knee set. She also had twitching in her eyes, a progressive neurological disease. Women need access to good medical care and not sloppy and ineffective care.*

Women's perception of their own social roles influences the importance they place on their own healthcare. Dialogues with NPs, PAs, and other health providers' help to educate these women while they struggle to provide care for others with their own co-morbidities. For the Medicaid population, in particular, the physician shortage is severe: many physicians will not accept Medicaid patients because of low reimbursements for their services and convoluted requirements for paperwork that must be filed with the state.[13] Women deserve far better treatment than they are currently receiving.

Wendy Grube: [During screening, I saw a] *woman with a Bartholin cyst, deep inside her labia.*[14] *I could sit and administer a little local anesthesia, drain her, and put her on some antibiotics. At least she would be okay for a while—but that is hit-and-run care, and I will not be around to follow up. What if she is not okay afterwards? What if she develops a sepsis? She is not going to be followed, and that is not good care. Some people say, "Well, that is better than nothing," but I am not so sure. She could apply hot compresses four times a day and the cyst will just open for her, but it has recurred over and over. She doesn't need a Band-Aid; she needs good care, and I cannot provide that. She has a problem that keeps coming back. There are these ethical dilemmas that you always run into.*

How Printed Aids Can Augment Oral Education

Southern people tell stories, often about themselves and their misadventures growing up and reaching adulthood. Women tell each other stories about their health concerns, and they learn from one another. Stories about illness and recovery can help others reach a higher understanding about cancer and cope with their own or a loved one's illness.

Many NPs say that it would be very useful to have access to brochures that they could use to educate their patients: "*We could say, 'These are your four big issues. Now I am going to sit down and talk to you about them.' Because we are teachers, we want to be able to explain to our patient how these four issues contribute to her overall health and how she can manage her symptoms. Educating patients is much better than saying, 'Okay, your blood pressure is high. No more salt, and get out and walk.'*"

One woman commented, "*I sit in the waiting room and think, oh, there are all these things wrong with me, and I don't really want to read all these brochures. However, I would listen if someone sat down with me and went over the materials.*" It is important that both healthcare professionals and community volunteers have some educational materials to give to the women they work with about some of the conditions the women have—something that the women can read on their own.

Women are given brochures on cervical cancer, breast cancer, hypertension, and diabetes, as well as other common health ailments. It is critical that someone the women trust, a friend who understands the information or a healthcare provider, be available to explain what she is reading. Informational brochures should show pictures and explain what the choices are if you or a loved one is diagnosed with the disease. Professional care providers are needed to clarify critical choices that must be made with regard to the disease, and then neighbors can back up the choices with their own stories. Providing choices for care is critical when confronting a debilitating illness, potential surgery, or even death.

Many of the women Wendy Grube and her NP and midwifery students see during screening have multiple medical complexities with several co-morbidities going on at once.

Wendy Grube: *With two clinicians in the room, we can learn more. I can see how other people manage the patient and what other nurses see that I might not see. We are all students and can learn from each other, especially if we are working together examining a patient. Even though you have some confidence in your skills, it is nice to go back and forth with someone who may have a different level of expertise. We could see more patients than if it had just been me as an individual. Patients are more satisfied with pairs and get better care as a result.*

Protecting Young Women

To protect tomorrow's women from cervical cancer, efforts to vaccinate girls and young women between ages 11 and 26 (before they become sexually active) against the human papillomavirus (HPV) need to be stepped up, despite the tremendous amount of effort that must go into training. Since the HPV vaccine campaign's launch in 2004, many bills on HPV and cervical cancer have been introduced across all 50 states.[15] The goal is to eradicate the disease. In the vast majority of cases, the virus causes no symptoms and will go away on its own.

Even though there is a lot of advertising about HPV and its relationship with cervical cancer, many younger women think that cervical cancer is a disease of older women—and that the vaccine is not for them. High-risk strains of HPV occur in 5 percent of women, and the American Cancer Society estimated that 11,070 women were impacted in 2008, with about 3,870 dying from HPV-related cancer. In conjunction with the Pap smear, the HPV test can be used with sexually active women to help detect the HPV virus.[16] The HPV test combined with the Pap smear is better at identifying women at risk for developing cervical cancer than the Pap smear alone. However, lack of insurance coverage continues to hamper efforts to ensure that all women have access to appropriate cervical cancer prevention and screening technology.

Many young Webster County women go out of the county to obtain birth control pills. It can be difficult to find practitioners who will prescribe the pill in this conservative, fundamentalist Christian region, so they travel to gynecologists on the other side of the mountains to safely obtain the pill.

How One Negative Experience Can Keep Women from Being Screened

One bad examination experience can sour a woman on medical care providers for the rest of her life. Some local women report having gone in for a Pap exam and, because they were obese or because they smoked or drank alcohol, having been berated so badly by the provider that they refused to return. Think about it:

> *You are told to take off your clothing and are stripped down to nothing. You are given this paper gown, told to lie on a metal table, and placed in a foreign environment with no control over your clothing. Then they put a paper drape over you and tell you to put your feet in the metal stirrups. You are treated as if you are nobody. I have seen male and female physicians doing pelvic exams who were so detached that they might as well have been working on a car.*

Appalachian men and women are proud, and they want to "take care of their own." Trust is the critical factor in people's acceptance of healthcare services, including prevention of, screening for, and treatment of cancer. If Appalachian women and men are to receive proper healthcare services, health professionals need to engage in positive communication with them. Health professionals need to understand how Appalachians face cancer and other illnesses and to develop a dialogue with them about how they can care for themselves and their families.

> *Nursing science goes beyond the provision of services to explore healthcare beliefs. We listen to and respect the concerns of community members and create collaborative efforts within their cultural context.*
>
> —Dr. Wendy Grube

Many of Wendy Grube's NPs want to help the patients they see during cancer screenings with primary care issues, but they are prevented from doing so because they will be leaving and cannot follow up. Here are some interchanges the NPs reported:

NP: *Do you have diabetes?*

Patient: *I think that is what I have pinpointed it to, but I really don't know.*

NP: *Do you have type one or type two diabetes?*

Patient: *I know that I do not take the shots.*

NP: *My patient had a blood pressure of 180 over 110, and I said to her, "Your blood pressure is rather high. Have you had any problems with your blood pressure in the past?" Well, the woman had had a procedure the year before, and the doctor had prescribed some medication—in fact, she had it in her purse. But she only took the pill every once in a while, when she was feeling really bad. She had no money—her husband had been laid off—and she wasn't going to take the medicine because she didn't think she could get it refilled.*

NP: *Why is it that almost every woman* [I see during screening] *has had a hysterectomy? I was surprised and a little bothered by that. Who is this doctor? A hysterectomy and a bladder tack all by the age of twenty-seven—and thirty years later she is still having hot flashes.*

Empowering Women through Positive Communication

Barriers to communication between locals and healthcare professionals include cultural differences and low health literacy. Honest and open dialogue between women and their healthcare providers is essential for establishing health goals, including those for cancer care. Healthcare providers need to be truthful with women about what is going on with them and to explain the options (both pros and cons) they have for care. It is important that care providers help women understand that they are the masters of their own fate and the captains of their own ship.

NP: *I saw two women who had lost more than thirty pounds by just taking soda out of their diet. It was empowering for them to hear me say, "You did that! You took control over your body. The choices that you made influenced your health." Their faces lit up. They were like, "Wow. I do have control. I did that—I made the choice to cut out soda, and I lost that weight. Great job!"*

Healthcare professionals carry a huge responsibility to both educate and listen. Each provider who passes on accurate information to a patient reinforces the stream of positive communication. Effective communication requires that the patient and the provider both understand one another and be understood by the other. Poor communication tends to produce mistakes and bad medical care. With lives at stake, healthcare professionals need to practice their communication skills: listen first, and then give advice.[17]

NPs can empower their patients through both open

communication and education. One NP empowered her female patients to participate in their own wellness by teaching them to examine their vaginas using mirrors. Another helped her patient understand the difference between the feel of a healthy thyroid and an unhealthy one. Shifting power to women for watching over their own bodies makes an incredible difference.

One NP told her patient: *This is your body. This is what we are looking at today. You haven't seen it in fifty-five years, but you will see it today. Feel this on your thyroid. This is not normal. Now feel mine. That* [information] *is empowering.* [The patient] *can now keep track of how her thyroid operates compared with mine.*

Another NP remarked: *It would be cool to bring a mirror for each exam room. Many of the women we work with don't know if they still have a cervix or if anything* [unusual] *is going on down there. With a mirror, they can look at their vagina and learn what is normal and what is not and be informed. Mirrors should be part of every exam.*

Social Justice Issues and Rural Health

Because access to cancer care in Appalachia remains limited, it is even more important that cancer control experts promote the value of cancer prevention, which includes regular screenings and changes in lifestyle. Rural residents need to understand that cancer control is feasible. Trust is critical to Appalachian women's acceptance of information and use of available health services, including screening and treatment for cancer. Positive communication between patients and their families and health professionals is instrumental in creating trust.

Wendy Grube to her NP students: *It is really easy when you are back in Philadelphia to forget about West Virginia. So, how do you go about making a change for these people?*

What are the little things that you can do to make a change in healthcare to positively impact how people conduct their lives? You already did it, just by being here. It was getting in, doing the screenings, and finding problems and bringing them to the attention of the WVBCCSP people. They pay attention to what you wrote in that little paragraph on the chart, and they will follow up. Also, just by talking with the patients you saw, you made them feel better.

How Dr. Grube Has Used Her Leadership Skills to Benefit Rural Women

In the six years that Wendy Grube and her NP students have been coming to Webster Springs, West Virginia, they have spent considerable time doing cancer screenings, examining women, and identifying cases of co-morbidity while at the same time avoiding "hit-and-run" care. In her work with the WVBCCSP, Wendy has displayed her leadership skills by:

- Understanding that shared personal stories of cancer experiences can impel rural women (and men) to seek cancer treatment, and that religious faith and effective cancer control can co-exist.

- Becoming involved with the Webster Springs community to better understand the sociocultural influences that affect reproductive healthcare and screening practices.

- Teaching her students how to treat rural women with sensitivity and how to truly listen to their concerns without judgment.

- Collaborating with rural women to identify their misperceptions of the facts about cervical and breast cancer and to shift their thinking to today's effective methods of screening and preventive care.

- Encouraging her NP students to empower the women they screen by talking with them about their concerns and providing education about altering their diets to improve their overall health or providing mirrors in the examining room.

- Providing accurate cancer information which open communication, changes in life style and use of available health services, such as the West Virginia Breast and Cervical Cancer Screening Program.

- Engaging rural women in dialogues about their options for care, including helping their family, friends, and neighbors by sharing accurate cancer screening information.

And most especially:

- Tirelessly returning twice a year, since 2006, to screen the women of Webster County for breast and cervical cancer.

Conclusion

States continue their efforts to make cervical cancer a disease that can be erased. Cervical cancer mortality rates continue to decline, and use of the HPV vaccine has major implications in the prevention of this disease. Cervical cancer screening, which includes the Pap test and HPV testing, is essential for women, as are regular physician checkups. According to Mary Brooks Beatty, president of Women in Government, *"This disease is almost completely preventable and we need to ensure that all women have access to the most appropriate cervical cancer prevention technologies, that socioeconomic status is not a barrier to receiving care, and that women around the world benefit from the tools that have helped make a difference in the battle against cervical cancer in the United States."*[18]

Screening mammograms can check for breast cancer in women who show no signs of the disease, and diagnostic mammograms check for lumps when other symptoms of the disease have been found. Results from randomized clinical trials show that screening mammography helps reduce the number of deaths from breast cancer among women aged 40–74. However, screening mammograms are also associated with the potential for harm when they identify "problems" that do not cause symptoms or threaten a woman's life but that require further exploration or treatment once identified. The National Cancer Institute recommends that women 40 and older should have screening mammograms every two years. Women younger than 40 years need a baseline mammogram, with additional screenings in their forties.[19]

Appalachia encompasses 406 counties in 13 states, ranging from New York to Mississippi. Across Appalachia, advanced-practice nurses conduct more Pap tests than anywhere else in the country and are responsible for finding more abnormal Pap results and treating the women involved. These screenings can have far-reaching consequences, as Wendy Grube notes:

If we are going to change the healthcare system and make it more effective, we need to talk about preventive care. [Screening] is really important and critical to the lives of these women. Recognize and value that what you are doing is saving lives, but [never forget] that we have to keep these women in the screening process.

Actions for Nurse Practitioners

Question

Only when women (and men) have up-to-date information about cancer can they receive the care they rightfully deserve. How can you encourage your patients to take cancer prevention steps (such as seeing that the young women in their lives are vaccinated against HPV) and to maintain timely routine screenings for cervical and breast cancer?

Using Community Forums to Convey Cancer Information

- Brainstorm ways to use focus groups to increase patients' knowledge about cancer prevention, screening, and treatment.
- Consider how you might involve your urban or rural clinic in providing social and emotional support for people living with cancer.

Example:

Though cancer support groups can be emotionally draining, their purpose is to bring people together to share their personal stories about cancer. No one should have to face cancer alone. Consider ways to use the power of your group to lift spirits and provide support. List ways in which you can use your own knowledge about cancer to educate others and to help group members talk to each other about how they are approaching their own care.

Balancing Faith and Cancer Control, and Building Trust

- List some approaches for combating distrust of physicians and hospitals among patients visiting rural and urban clinics.
- Instead of automatically rejecting an individual's religious

belief, engage in problem solving to address the person's concerns about receiving cancer care.

Example:

Distrust of the medical establishment is higher in minority and rural communities because of personal and family experiences with providers who were perceived as incompetent, motivated by profit, or judgmental. What steps can you take to engage in honest dialogues about health options with your patients? What teaching approaches might be successful in encouraging them to undergo preventive screenings?

Empowering Women to Take Charge of Their Own Health Care

- The long-term goal of choosing a healthy diet is to have more energy and to reduce the risk of cancer and other diseases.
- Drinking lots of water helps us stay hydrated and flushes wastes and toxins from our systems.

Example:

When women see that something as simple as cutting soda from their diet can result in a thirty-pound weight loss, they discover that they can make a difference in their own health. Encourage your patients to make healthy food choices. List ways in which you can encourage your patients to eat right, get enough exercise, and pay attention to their own mental health. People often mistake thirst for hunger; staying hydrated reduces feelings of tiredness and low energy.

Getting Enough Exercise

- Find some sort of activity that you like to do and do it every day such as walking, biking, yoga, weight lifting, or aerobics. Exercise is motivating.
- Improving your physical health by taking care of your body increases your mental and emotional health and well-being.

Example:

Childhood obesity is a growing global concern, and physical exercise may help reduce the impact of both child and adult obesity. Frequent exercise protects and boosts the immune system, prevents chronic diseases, and prevents heart disease, type 2 diabetes, and depression. Exercise helps us maintain a positive self-image and should be done regularly.

Encouraging Appropriate Screenings

- Medically disadvantaged patients can find good healthcare in public health programs, community clinics, and school-based programs.
- Tie Pap tests, mammograms, cholesterol tests, blood pressure checks, and smoking cessation and weight loss counseling to your patients' health improvement goals.

Example:

Work with your patients to address their most pressing health concerns. Focus on common diseases for which there are accurate screening tests and effective treatments, such as diabetes testing, heart monitoring, and asthma control. Physicians routinely subject their patients to tests that are unnecessary and not recommended by any major North American clinical organization. Work with your patients to help them identify the steps they can take to improve their health and get better care for their health problems.

CHAPTER FIVE

Retail Clinics: Expansion of the Nurse Practitioner Role into Primary Care

Primary care remains the lynchpin of high-performing healthcare: preventive care maintained throughout peoples' lives increase life expectancy. Evidence shows that healthcare that employs a strong primary care model results in better health and overall well-being.[1] People need primary care providers who have knowledge of their health issues and who see them as individuals. However, the American Academy of Family Physicians predicts a shortfall of 40,000 primary care providers by 2020, and for many patients, the average waiting time to see a physician for non-urgent care can exceed 90 days.[2] This type of holding pattern should not exist; patients need to be able to enter the healthcare system, be seen in a reasonable amount of time, and know that their needs are being addressed.

Nurse practitioners (NPs) can help fill the current gap by performing many of the tasks now done by family physicians and other primary care providers. Retail clinics employing NPs and physician assistants (PAs) are providing treatment and evaluation for a limited number of conditions at lower cost than, but with quality comparable to, physician offices, urgent care clinics, and emergency departments. Likewise, the ongoing increases in medical costs are unsustainable and unsupportable. According to a new Census Bureau report, people aged 65 or older now make up 13 percent of the U.S. population.[3] There were 40.3 million people aged 65 and older on April 1, 2010, up 5.3 percent from 35 million in 2000 (and just 3.1 million in 1900). Although seniors are getting older and sicker with age-related diseases, they continue to have high expectations for receiving quality healthcare at reasonable prices. Retail clinics, also called convenient care clinics (CCCs), offer one solution to rising health costs. When NPs and PAs work collaboratively with physicians and other healthcare professionals, they can provide coordinated high-quality care at substantially reduced fees.[4]

You are never too old to set another goal or to dream a new dream

An Early Retail Clinic Model

Sandra Ryan, MSN, CPNP, FCPP, FAANP, is the chief nurse practitioner officer for Take Care Health Systems' (TCHS) Consumer Solutions Group (CSG) Walgreens, overseeing clinical and operational leadership nationally. In addition, she works closely with Walgreens' chief medical officer in areas such as clinical governance, clinical research, and quality initiatives. Sandra is one of six founding officers of Take Care Health Systems, the first chief nurse practitioner officer in the retail industry, and a founding board member of the Convenient Care Association (CCA), a national association of retail clinic companies.

Take Care Health Systems initially limited its scope of clinical services and entered the marketplace as an acute care, self-limiting company, meaning that clinic staff saw only a handful of diagnostic codes. At that time, it was the right strategy, because retail clinics were meeting with resistance and apprehension from the American Medical Association and from insurers, who did not really understand the model.

From the beginning, TCHS has been a very open company, willing to listen to a variety of ideas. Its leaders understand the fine balance between meeting business needs and also meeting colleagues' and patients' needs. The company values relationships and lets staff know that their opinions count; in fact, relationships form the basis for what leadership calls *our secret sauce.* The TCHS model centers on the patient, aiming to make patients happy with their care, pleased with the results, and on the road to recovery.

What the Walgreens Acquisition Has Meant for Take Care

In 2007, within two years of Take Care's founding, Walgreens acquired Take Care Health Systems and soon after doubled its size from five markets and approximately 50 clinics to 360 clinics in nineteen states. Walgreens' leaders were committed to the vision and mission of Take Care and appreciative of the great culture and values of TCHS. Quality and compassionate care would remain at the core of patient treatment as Walgreens and Take Care looked to revolutionize healthcare together. Take Care retail clinics are at select Walgreens, located near the pharmacy where they provide services to prevent, treat, and manage health concerns. Board-certified family NPs and PAs listen to patients' needs, conduct thorough examinations, and provide individualized diagnoses and treatment plans.[5] Pressed for time, most primary care physicians cannot afford to spend extra time with each patient, whereas NPs can provide longer consultations and education. Consequently, NPs have consistently high patient satisfaction scores, and nurses are consistently rated by the Gallup organization as one of the most trusted professionals.

With the transition from a small, standalone organization to part of the much larger Walgreens, Take Care Clinics' healthcare providers worried that their relationship with Sandra would become more distant and difficult. To maintain the earlier closeness and to help new TCHS providers get to know the "real" Sandra, she blogs, incorporating information about her family life into her postings. Sharing pictures and notes about her family, her vacations, and her life with the 1,300 NPs under her leadership helps reinforce her human side and also helps her gain the trust of her NP staff and healthcare providers. This is especially important in a company like TCHS, with numerous clinics in nineteen states across the country.

Consumer Access to Retail Clinics

Eighty-eight percent of retail clinics (Take Care, CVS MinuteClinics, Kroger's, and Target) are located in major cities, and one-third of the U.S. patient population can find a clinic close to their homes.[6] Most retail clinics operate in those areas of large cities that have lower poverty rates and higher median incomes. Twenty-nine percent of the population lives within a ten-minute drive of a retail clinic. Currently, there are more than 1,350 CCCs throughout the United States, and most are open seven days a week: twelve hours a day Monday through Friday and eight hours on the weekends. Because CCCs are new, only a small percentage of people receive their healthcare in the retail setting; however, it is estimated that the number will grow dramatically in the future.[7] More than one in three consumers are receptive to using retail clinics, and interest in retail clinics is especially high among baby boomers and young adults.

In terms of the TCHS Walgreens retail chain, 75 percent of all Americans live within five miles of a Walgreens drug store, giving TCHS the ability to open clinics in locations convenient to potential healthcare consumers. Its ability to expand beyond its current footprint in fewer than half the U.S. states should prime it for future growth.

Comparing the Cost of Care in Various Healthcare Clinics

With healthcare costs extremely high, anything that retail clinics can do to help promote health, prevent disease, or treat problems early on can improve both health and financial outcomes for patients and the healthcare system. But the larger story is that CCCs across the United States are providing equal-quality healthcare with lower costs than emergency rooms, urgent care center, or primary care physicians.

Convenient Care Clinics vs. Take Care Clinics

- Health Affairs study shows that approximately $4.4 billion a year in unnecessary Emergency Room visits could be saved by utilizing retail clinics and urgent care clinics instead.

- According to a Gallup study, Take Care Health ranks among the top 10% of all organizations globally in engaging customers.

In one study, claims data from 2005 to 2006 for treating three acute illnesses—otitis media (middle ear infection), pharyngitis (inflammation of the throat), and urinary tract infection (UTI)— were aggregated into care episodes, including initial and follow-up visits, pharmaceuticals, and ancillary tests. After 2,100 episodes of care for patients treated in a retail clinic were identified, the episodes were matched with those of patients treated at a physician's office, urgent care center, or emergency department. The cost of care was 30–40 percent lower at a retail clinic than at a physician's office or an urgent care center and 80 percent lower than at an emergency department.[8] Lower rates for laboratory testing, patient evaluation, and management visits accounted for the largest price differentials. Retail clinics provided the same quality of care for these three common illnesses as the other venues, but at substantially lower fees.

Approximately one in five visits to a primary care physician and one in ten visits to an emergency department can be taken care of at a retail clinic for less money. It is estimated that reducing emergency department visits for non-emergency care could save $4.4 billion annually.[9] The current healthcare system cannot sustain continued increases in the number of emergency room visits. Instead of the emergency department, healthcare consumers need to be encouraged to seek out urgent care centers and retail clinics for non-emergency care. Patient-centered care with a focus on quality and compassion keeps costs under control and increases patient satisfaction at retail clinics.

Profile of a Typical Retail Clinic Patient

CCCs typically serve patients lacking access to primary care health services. These patients seek out retail clinics for treatment of straightforward problems because they value convenience: the ability to walk in, sign in at the kiosk, and be seen relatively quickly.

Members of the Convenient Care Association (CCA), a national association of retail clinic companies, were invited to participate in a national study on retail-clinic patient sex, age, and method of payment for the visit and whether the patient had a primary care physician (PCP).[10] Forty-three percent of retail clinic patients tend to be young adults, aged 18–44. Two-thirds of retail patients have health insurance; the remaining third pay in cash. Retail clinics focus on a small set of clinical complaints: ten complaints account for 90 percent of all clinic visits. Concerns have been raised that retail clinics disrupt primary care relationships; however, three-fifths of retail clinic patients do not have a PCP, so there is no relationship to disrupt. Another concern is coordination of care and communication with physicians' offices. At any time, patients can request a printed summary of their clinic visit and have it faxed to their physician's office.

Visiting a Retail Clinic

At Take Care Clinics[SM], we believe providing
quality care starts with having compassionate,
expert healthcare providers.

A young adult patient walks into a Walgreens and finds the retail clinic in the back of the store, near the pharmacy. The patient may have heard about the clinic from someone else or may have found it by Googling "walk-in-clinic." The patient signs in at the kiosk. Currently Take Care Clinics' hours of operation are 8 a.m. to 8 p.m. Monday through Friday and 9:30 a.m. to 5 p.m. on weekends. The clinics are closed only two days of the year, Christmas and Thanksgiving. Generally the day after those or other holidays, such as Easter Sunday, is extremely busy. Seasonality has a direct impact on the number of patients seeking out retail clinics. The clinics tend to show increased volume during cold and flu season, and clinic volume picks up for school physicals, immunizations, flu shots, and the allergy season. When physicians' offices are busy and unable to accept patients, clinic volume goes up as well. Retail clinics are seen as a complement to the current healthcare system and play a needed role in access to care.

Growth of the NP's Role in Primary Care

NPs may play an even greater role in the future as primary care providers. With the looming shortage of primary care physicians, twenty-eight states currently have granted prescriptive authority to NPs and PAs.[11] With 32 million Americans scheduled to gain health insurance by 2014, NPs will need to play a bigger role in the care of routine illnesses. Nurse-managed clinics are seeing increased funding. The U.S. Department of Health and Human Services announced on May 2, 2012, that 400 community health centers will be getting a $728 million boost to build, renovate, and improve operations. The money is intended to pay for increased preventive care targeting the chronically ill. Expected to serve 1.3 million patients, most of these clinics will be led by NPs and PAs.[12]

NPs and PAs are board certified and highly educated practitioners who are licensed to treat both acute and chronic illnesses, order lab tests and x-rays, and write prescriptions. In the retail setting they are currently treating a limited number of common illnesses and providing preventive care using evidence-based guidelines and their clinical judgment. To ensure quality and consistency in this new healthcare model, CCA developed quality and safety standards for the industry. CCA's quality and safety standards far exceed those recommended by the American Medical Association, the American Academy of Family Practitioners, and the American Academy of Pediatrics. CCA members are committed to monitoring quality on an ongoing basis through peer reviews, collaborating physician reviews, collecting and reporting data on quality and safety standards, and monitoring patient satisfaction, which generally exceeds 90 percent.[13]

Retail clinics offer high-quality care and relieve overburdened physician offices and emergency rooms while increasing access to care. Making better use of advanced practice nurses needs to be front and center in any healthcare reform package.[14] Integrating the healthcare workforce—primary care physicians, NPs, PAs, and specialists—into healthcare teams should improve the health of all those in the system and ultimately decrease cost to the system.

Job projections for NPs and PAs continue to grow in both primary care and specialty settings. The U.S. Bureau of Labor Statistics predicts that from 2008 to 2018, there will be a 23 percent increase in nursing jobs and a 41 percent increase in PA jobs.[15] The combined NP/PA workforce will then be 75 percent as large as the physician workforce in both primary care and specialty settings. NPs and PAs will play an important role in remedying such healthcare challenges as impending physician shortages, a growing aging population, and healthcare reform, and they will serve on the front lines in the fight against chronic illnesses such as cancer, heart conditions, and diabetes.

Unfortunately, many states continue to maintain barriers that prevent NPs and PAs from providing the breadth of care for which their training qualifies them. States vary as to what they allow NPs and PAs to do.[16] For example:

- In Florida and Alabama, NPs cannot prescribe narcotics.

- In Washington, NPs can recommend medical marijuana.

- In Montana, NPs need not have physician participation, but many other states put physicians in charge of NPs or require a collaborative agreement signed by a physician.

TCHS currently operates only in states that require collaborative agreements with physicians. The goal for its clinics and NP staff is to provide the best quality of care for patients in collaboration with the healthcare community in which the clinics operate. At the grassroots level, TCHS believes collaboration among healthcare professionals is the key to better patient outcomes and more satisfied colleagues. Collaborating physicians and TCHS NPs are a team. NPs can call collaborating physicians with questions anytime during clinic hours, because the physicians are on call to support the NPs. One profession cannot render all care, but a fully functioning healthcare team made up of NPs, physicians, specialists, and other healthcare members can. Team care provides patients with expertise and services that coordinate all aspects of their healthcare, from a sore throat requiring attention that can be delivered by an NP in a retail clinic setting through difficult or chronic conditions requiring an extensive evaluation by a physician or a specialist's care received in a traditional setting or hospital.

Businesses and other organizations are focusing more attention on delivery of healthcare in the retail setting. These entities have increased their support for legislative changes to rectify inconsistencies in state scope of practice laws, which define nurse roles, outline oversight requirements, and articulate prescriptive authority regulations. State-to-state differences make it difficult for retail operators to manage each state's practice requirements. State regulations can be unduly restrictive, costly, and impose barriers to patient care by keeping NPs from providing the comprehensive primary care permitted by their licenses and education.

Best Practice Standards and TCHS's NPs

TCHS has policies and clinical guidelines to support the 1,300 NPs at its 360 clinics. The company promotes evidence-based practice and identifies and executes best practice standards across all its sites. However, TCHS believes that its colleagues should be able to utilize their clinical judgment and education when delivering care. If an NP decides to choose a treatment path that differs from the clinical guideline, she must document the reason for the deviation from what is considered best practice. TCHS gives its NPs tools to make good decisions, but also allows them the freedom to make appropriate choices based on the patient's needs. TCHS recognizes that its NPs must have the freedom to make independent clinical decisions because medicine is not black or white or an exact science; it is more of an art, and there is a lot of gray in between.

TCHS is guideline driven, unlike other competing retail clinic chains, which are protocol driven. A protocol-driven model does not permit nurses to step outside the boundaries. In a guideline-driven model, the guidelines are there to *"assist nurse practitioners in making decisions."*

Sandra Ryan: *My son was ten years old and had a sore throat. He had a high fever, was flushed in the face, had palpable enlarged nodes on his neck, exudate on his throat, and was nauseous. He smelled like strep and was dry heaving. At the time, [TCHS] did not have clinics where I live, so I took him to one of our competitors. At ten years old, he was a big, strong kid and would gag every time the nurse practitioner tried to do a strep test on him. According to the clinical criteria, he had strep. In our company, the nurse practitioner would have the ability to document, "Attempted throat culture twice. Patient uncooperative. Based on all the clinical symptoms and evaluation, patient has clinical strep," and to treat him accordingly.*

In this competitor's environment, the nurse was not able to do that. She said to me, "I can check that his test was positive, and then the system will let me go ahead and write you a script." She was willing to compromise her own integrity and her practice to take care of one patient. She was not thinking that she was putting herself and her credentials at risk because she wanted to take care of my son.

You need to be able to let the NPs practice to the ability level of their education and training. Give them the tools, guidelines, and support to help them make good clinical decisions about care.

Increasing Education Regarding Antibiotics

In her leadership role, Sandra analyzes data to see how the TCHS NPs are doing compared with their peers. For example, one assessment is how they score on HEDIS (Healthcare Effectiveness Data and Information Set) measures compared with industry-wide results.

In a recent study of treatment of acute pharyngitis in a retail setting, the rates of adherence to a practice guideline were measured as one indicator of clinical quality. Of 57,331 patient visits for evaluation of acute pharyngitis, 39,530 cases had negative rapid strep test results, and NPs and PAs adhered to the guidelines by withholding unnecessary antibiotics in more than 99 percent of those cases. Of the 13,471 patients with a positive rapid strep test, 99.75 percent received appropriate antibiotics.[17]

Bronchitis is usually a viral infection, and NPs should not prescribe antibiotics for its treatment because they generally do more harm than good, especially when there is a concern about antibiotic resistance. Within TCHS, 50 percent of patients with bronchitis do not get an antibiotic. A year ago, the TCHS bronchitis scores were pretty comparable to those of the external community—that is, to the national benchmark of three in four receiving an antibiotic. TCHS leadership determined that that was not good enough and traveled to clinics in all nineteen states to provide staff education. Leadership firmly believes that what gets measured gets done. Accordingly, educators worked with the NPs and PAs at all Take Care Clinics to make sure that everyone understood that bronchitis is a viral infection. They showed staff HEDIS protocols and national benchmark standards. As a result, benchmark scores improved significantly. This is good news, especially when the statistics are used to show other key stakeholders, such as physician groups and managed care organizations, the value of retail clinics in promoting health.

TCHS leadership knows that it is difficult for their NPs to say no when the patient is insisting, *"I need an antibiotic, and my doctor gave me one last year."* NPs know why these patients think they need antibiotics, but there are evidence-based reasons why prescribing them is not good practice. TCHS's NPs share with their patients the facts about the increased prevalence of resistance to antibiotics and the body's inability to fight off further infections. The NPs empower their patients with handouts, talking points, and follow-up phone calls on their illness, and they set clear expectations for their patients. They instruct them that a viral illness will take five to seven days to run its course. They tell patients that they will feel better soon, but that they will not feel better tomorrow.

> The major reason we are seeing antibiotic resistance is overuse of antibiotics in the population for illnesses that don't require antibiotics—typically colds, sore throats, "bronchitis"—illnesses that would resolve themselves because they are caused by viruses.
>
> —Bob Harrison

TCHS's Expansion of Services

Quality and compassionate caring form the core of the Take Care Health System. TCHS clinics measure consumer satisfaction through Gallup polls. The company ranks among the top 10 percent of all organizations globally for engaging patients. All patients who come to a TCHS clinic receive a follow-up call from a health professional within 48 hours of their visit, to check on how well they were treated

From my time in Health I know that choice empowers people's lives.
—John Hutton

As noted earlier, when it first opened its retail clinics, TCHS limited its scope of services. That was the right decision initially, but the company later recognized that it was not the right choice for the future. To maximize the benefits it was providing to patients, TCHS decided to expand its scope of services to include preventive screenings, immunizations, and specialty medication administration, and to look to chronic care. Its retail clinics now are providing patients with preventive screening services designed to identify chronic conditions or prevent catastrophic events, a needed focus for patients.

Patients are looking to the retail clinic to provide more primary care services. Evidence supports the fact that patient health outcomes are similar whether an NP or a physician treats them; however, patient satisfaction is higher among those seeing NPs. A study published in 2011[18] found that the care provided to patients by NPs and certified nurse midwives in collaboration with physicians was similar to (and sometimes better than) that provided by physicians alone. NPs had longer consultations, provided more patient training, and spent longer periods of time with patients than physicians did. Research suggests that between 25 and 70 percent of care currently done by physicians could be switched to NPs with no loss in quality and patient satisfaction.[19]

NPs now represent about 9 percent of all nurses, and their numbers continue to grow. Moving into more chronic care treatment and management represents the next step for these highly educated professionals. NPs can help fill the gap of primary care formerly provided by primary care physicians, freeing primary care physicians to attend to the more complicated illnesses formerly requiring a specialist's attention. Utilizing healthcare professionals to their highest level of education and training will help enable us to meet the needs of our patients today and in the future.

Some Examples of Compassionate Care

A customer looking for Benadryl walked into a Walgreens store that happened to have a Take Care Clinic. Inside the store, the gentleman fainted, fell to the floor, and could not talk. The NP ran to the front of the Walgreens to help the man; at that moment, the market manager, a licensed NP, happened to walk into the store. The two recognized that the man was having an anaphylactic reaction and needed epinephrine immediately. They injected him with an EpiPen and called the emergency number and got him to a hospital, where he received further medical attention. A month later, the man returned to thank the NP and the market manager for saving his life. Recorded by the store's video camera, the actions of the staff showed the nurses' care, compassion, and quick clinical intervention in treating the man until the ambulance arrived. The staff's concern, attentiveness, and keen judgment kept this gentleman alive.

At a Texas Walgreens on a holiday weekend, a woman complained to the pharmacist that she was not feeling well. The pharmacist said, *"We have a clinic right here."* The woman signed in at the kiosk for care. She told the NP, *"I called my provider's office and told them I was not feeling well; they told me to come in next week."* The NP took the time to question the woman, who was over fifty, thoroughly about her symptoms. The woman complained of feeling dizzy, being diaphoretic, and experiencing extreme fatigue. The patient was not obese, nor was she a smoker, but based on her comments about how she was feeling, the NP said, *"I think you have heart disease."*

The NP triaged the woman to the hospital, where she was able to receive the level of care she needed for her heart condition. The clinicians at the emergency room said, *"The nurse practitioner who treated you saved you from a stroke or a heart attack."* Six months later, the woman emailed Sandra Ryan about first being ignored by her physician and then being questioned by the NP regarding her heart. She wanted to thank the NP for the compassionate care that she had received that holiday weekend.

Importance of the Electronic Medical Record

TCHS's proprietary electronic medical record (EMR) process allows collaborating community physicians to review a percentage of a clinic's records and give feedback on the quality of care the NPs at the clinic are providing. The EMR also allows NPs to review de-identified peer records across TCHS's 360 clinics. Everything entered into the EMR can be mined for data reporting. Quality is measured using traditional indicators such as patient wait times, length of the patient's visit, patient engagement, and appropriate antibiotic prescribing.

The goal is to provide an exceptional patient experience, so many things are measured to make sure that patients are being seen in a reasonable amount of time, are receiving quality care, and are happy with the service they receive. As a model of walk-in care, the clinics have to focus on patient convenience and the flow of patient care. EMR technology allows patient health data, genetic makeup, and other personal information to be used to help predict the health challenges patients may face.[20] TCHS makes use of electronic kiosks, electronic records, and electronic prescribing. Management can track everything from patient complaints, to patient compliments, to incident reports, to quality scores, all electronically.

Joyce Komori, clinical operations manager for TCHS, is responsible for translating medical practice requirements into information technology language to facilitate the development of a proprietary EMR that meets the needs of TCC's care providers. Nursing traditionally has relied on paper on clipboards for patient information; making the transition from paper to an EMR system can be challenging. The change requires a mental shift, and managing through the change is not always easy. Training is required to help the NPs learn the EMR system, to remove barriers, and to get NPs comfortable with the use of computers. Even with training, the transition is not always smooth: nurses cannot always find what they are looking for, or feel comfortable without paper files.

EMR technology offers important benefits to physicians and to retail clinic staff. Transferring paper records to an EMR allows the staff to operate more efficiently. With an EMR, every workstation becomes a chart rack; there are fewer lost charts, less time is spent filing, and there is universal access to charts. It is easier to comply with chart requests; accordingly, there is improved external communication and fewer callbacks from pharmacies. EMRs contain built-in protocols and reminders, can improve medication management, can foster consistent patient communication, and can help staff engage patients more actively in their own healthcare.

Committing to the Underserved

Retail clinics tend not to be located in medically underserved neighborhoods. In a recent census tract of 914 clinics, only 14 percent served the poor. That said, TCHS promotes its intent to provide high quality, low-cost, accessible healthcare to all communities.

Community health centers serve neighborhoods in urban and rural areas and serve low-income people. The U.S. Department of Health and Human Services Secretary, Kathleen Sebelius, has said, *"For many Americans, community health centers are the major source of care that ranges from prevention to treatment of chronic diseases."*[21] Since 2009, employment at community health centers has increased by 15 percent. However, it can be difficult for patients to complete the maze of paperwork required before the first visit. Options for clinical care remain tightly controlled, with few sources available between community health centers and retail clinics. Often, a retail clinic is the best bet for low-cost health care.

Sue Ferbet, Regional Vice President, Northeast Region: *We are the less-cost alternative for that working individual who has no insurance. One of the questions that we ask patients* at our clinics is, "How did you hear about us?" I asked this question of a gentleman I saw while I was working in one of our clinics. The man responded, "I was referred from County Health. I needed to be seen for a sinus infection, and they told me it would be cheaper here. I have a job, I make a decent living, and I just do not have health insurance." Because [the county health clinic charges on] a sliding scale, their cost was more than ours. Also, to get into a lot of the county health clinics, the amount of paperwork and the time you have to wait also play a role. If you are sick today, you don't want to wait three weeks to get into the system. Even though the community health clinics are federally funded, the funding must come through the states. It is not all equal, unfortunately.

We Are NP Leaders

Sue Ferbet: We try to promote from within. Patricia Jacob is a great example. She was a clinician in one of our clinics, and now she is a manager of a market. All of us [managers] are able to fill in at any of the clinics. I am licensed and credentialed and can work in any of the Missouri clinics with a collaborating physician. Patty can work in either the Delaware or our Pennsylvania clinics because she lives in Delaware and manages our Pennsylvania clinics. She can fill in whenever she is needed. There is a lot more respect and acceptance for our leadership because the NPs know we can do the job that they are doing and understand that we "get it."

Because we are all NPs (with a few PAs in some of our markets), it promotes our profession. Most of us were RNs first for a number of years and then went on to pursue additional degrees, not because someone told us to, but because that is the way we are wired. Many of us are very active in legislative *issues and in our professional organizations. We are very attuned to our profession and to making sure that people understand who and what we are. None of us stands alone. We are all in this together and want to make a difference to our profession and how others view our credentials.*

One Nurse's Leadership Accomplishments

Sandra Ryan has done so much to promote the value and recognition of NPs within TCHS's Take Care clinics, Walgreens and the retail industry. She has been recognized by numerous institutions for her leadership and commitment to advancing the role of the NP and for her commitment to improving healthcare nationally. Sandra:

- Driven investor interest and value as a founder of a venture-backed enterprise, culminating in the sale of Take Care Health to Walgreens in 2007. This was the largest industry transaction in the healthcare space at the time.

- Led start-up operations through periods of rapid growth, managing resources, ensuring excellence in quality and execution, expanding revenue, and increasing profitability year over year.

- Established and cultivated a system of NP leadership for an evolving industry, authorizing operational-clinical leadership teams of nurse practitioners, medical assistants, and collaborating physicians.

- Introduced a patient-centric care approach, initiating 24- to 48-hour callbacks for all patients and establishing the courtesy call as an added benefit that differentiates Walgreens from similar health and wellness models and focuses on customer relations.

- Contributed materially to the development of technological support, which is crucial to the successful creation of a proprietary EMR system from a healthcare provider perspective.

- Spearheaded creation and implementation of a proprietary EMR quality assurance and risk management program, with data available and reportable for all providers and clinics at all levels nationally.

- Instituted evidence-based practice standards leading to HEDIS consistently exceeding 90 percent of national standards.

- Promoted clinical guidelines for NP practice and the use of clinical judgment.

- Achieved outstanding patient engagement results, with TCHS's Take Care Clinics ranking in the top 10 percent of the Gallup organization database nationally. Results show that Take Care Clinics engage more than three out of every four patients.

- Served as Walgreens' representative on the board of the Convenient Care Association and chair for both the Provider Task Force and the Clinical Advisory Committee.

- Led development and implementation of the Convenient Care Association's industry-wide Quality and Safety Standards, a third party certification process for the retail industry, and initiated the Retail Education Congress for practitioners.

- Is a nationally sought-out speaker on retail clinics and NP leadership.

Conclusion

More than ten million American families receive care from 1,350 retail clinics across America. These retail clinics are staffed primarily with NPs and PAs. Since the 1960s, NPs have also grown community health centers to more than 7,354 sites across the country, providing care to more than 16 million patients.[22] The collective experience of retail clinics like CVS's Minute Clinics, Walgreens's Take Care Clinics, Kroger's, and Target speaks to the role of the NP in the evolution of 21st century healthcare. Healthcare consumers are gaining a basic understanding of what NPs can do and the legitimacy of their credentials.

In universities across America, NP enrollment is steadily increasing, and salaries for those with NP degrees are going up. Yet nursing schools face severe budget constraints and cannot accommodate the thousands of well-qualified nurses seeking further education. The impact of these individuals' inability to receive the training they desire will be felt by all patients. The nursing workforce faces losing more than 500,000 nurses to retirement, a number that simply cannot be ignored. Universities must step up the training of NPs, despite the fact that within the next ten years, half of the U.S. nursing school faculty will reach retirement age. A pool of advanced degree nurses will be needed to respond to the growing population of insured and uninsured Americans looking for affordable and effective healthcare.

Actions for Nurse Practitioners

Question for Reflection

What is your long-term vision for retail healthcare? How can NPs and PAs substitute for primary care physicians in the coming years so that PCPs can do more of the work now handled by specialists, and specialists can reserve their services for intricate care of the very ill?

Expanding the Role of NPs and PAs

- NPs and PAs may play an even greater role in the future as primary care providers.
- Retail clinics offer high-quality care for a limited number of common illnesses and provide preventive care using evidence-based guidelines.

Example:

NPs and PAs are board-certified, highly educated practitioners who can relieve overburdened primary care physicians and emergency rooms while increasing access to care. In terms of the quality and safety standards it has established, the Convenient Care Association (CCA) far exceeds those recommended by the American Medical Association, American Academy of Family Practitioners, and the American Academy of Pediatrics. How can you provide the right care at the right time for your patients?

Serving the Typical CCC Patient

- The patient typically is an adult, between the ages of 18 and 44. Two-thirds of retail clinic patients have health insurance; the rest pay in cash.
- An added benefit of a visit to some retail clinics is a courtesy call that is initiated within 24–48-hours of the visit.

Example:
Concerns have been raised that retail clinics may disrupt primary care relationships; however, three-fifths of retail clinic patients do not have a PCP. Another concern is the coordination of care with physician offices; however, at any time patients can request a printed summary of their clinic visit. Some retail providers have initiated telephone calls to all clinic patients between 24 and 48 hours after they are seen, to follow up and ensure that patients were satisfied with their care.

Empowering Others

- Develop relationships with patients so that they understand that you are invested in their care.
- Provide more health advice through brochures, training tips, and handouts.

Example:
Bring good data to the table, and let patients make educated decisions about their own care. Provide plenty of advice, training, and handouts to help patients choose between care options. One NP cited as an example her intervention with urinary incontinence in older women. She saw this condition as an opportunity to help women help themselves without surgery or drugs by teaching them simple things that they can do on their own to avoid aggressive treatment.

Listening to Patients

- Longer consultations lead to higher patient satisfaction. Learn to tune in to your patients for a true understanding of their needs.
- Patients may come in for a general physical and end up telling you that something else is bothering them. Truly listen, and follow their lead.

Example:

Nurse-led healthcare is associated with higher levels of patient satisfaction, longer consultations, screening, assessments, counseling, and patient follow-up. Patients seeing NPs received better care with no differences in patient outcomes. What you learn by listening carefully to your patients can be more valuable than the physical exam findings. You may need to advocate for the patient's right to care with primary care physicians who lack the time to administer or order the tests the patient needs.

Displaying Integrity

- Build trust by genuinely understanding the needs and priorities of your patients.
- Recognize that patients perceive healthcare professionals who sit down while listening as spending three times longer with them than when the professional stands.

Example:

Consistency of care is a critical healthcare component. In retail clinics, NPs develop trust by establishing relationships with the women and men in their community. As that trust builds, people come back to continue their care with the NPs who have shown understanding of and responsiveness to their healthcare needs.

CHAPTER SIX

School Health Centers: Empowering Students and Parents to Control Their Health Choices

Jonnie Hamilton, RN, MS, CPNP, CNA, is a nurse practitioner (NP) at Marcus Garvey Academy in Detroit and a recognized expert in pediatric care. More skilled than registered nurses, NPs can write prescriptions; order and read diagnostic tests; and diagnose and treat chronic conditions such as diabetes, high blood pressure, and asthma. In addition to clinical care, NPs address health promotion, disease prevention, and health education. They counsel and help schoolchildren (and often their families) make wise choices for healthy living.

With access to ongoing healthcare, recovering children in schools across the country can return to their classrooms on the same day or certainly within a week of diagnosis, whereas students without access to school health centers may have to stay home with similar illnesses. According to the National Assembly on School-Based Health Care, more than two thousand schools serving nearly 1.7 million children across the country have school-based health centers. Nationally, 24 percent of school-based health centers offer care to people living within the community, and 42 percent offer care to relatives of students.[1] Because of NP education and counseling, these healthcare consumers have fewer emergency room visits, shorter hospitals stays, and lower medication expenses.

Opening the Center, Reviewing Regulations, and Completing School Physicals

Jonnie Hamilton joined Marcus Garvey Academy in 1996; previously she held a position at the Detroit Medical Center (DMC) as director of education. As a pediatric nurse practitioner, Jonnie feels strongly about caring for and educating these school-aged children. Mr. Jordan, the urban school's long-time principal until his retirement in 2000, worked with Sister Mary Ellen Howard to find an NP who could set up the school-based clinic they both envisioned. The State of Michigan required proof that the school, with Jonnie in place, could open the health center, comply with all pertinent policies and procedures, complete patient records, complete school physicals, and train the students in chronic disease control. Jonnie came to talk to Sister Mary Ellen and promised to stay at the center for just two years—she has now been there for seventeen years.

Finding space for the school health center was the first hurdle. The selected site was previously a woodshop, and a lot of work went into bringing it up to code. Jonnie told the architects that she needed a bathroom, two treatment rooms, some storage space, and private offices for the therapist and the NP. The architects listened carefully and collaborated to give the health center everything it needed.

The first year was extremely hard because everything had to be created from nothing. Sister Mary Ellen is both a nurse and executive director of St. Francis Cabrini Clinic and has lots of experience working with health centers serving adults. She proved a huge help to Jonnie, assisting her in getting the basics completed to meet the State of Michigan's requirements. Policy basics included how the center would do lab work, deal with waste disposal, and comply with the many Occupational Safety and Health Administration (OSHA) regulations. Jonnie and Sister Mary Ellen rolled up their sleeves and read up on the requirements for a health center, studied the policy basics, and brought themselves up-to-date on the latest regulations. They also had to identify the limitations to the health services the center could provide and address such issues as collaborating with physicians and sending students to the emergency room when it was clear that the health center could not handle the patient's medical issues.

During that first year, the students needed to take school physical exams, including skin tests for tuberculosis. With 600 children in the school, the health center had to administer 150 school physical exams during the first year of operation, or about 25 percent of the total student body. Students from the sixth through eighth grades formed the first target group. When a new class of sixth graders enters the school, each student must complete a school physical; classes usually contain 30–35 students (for a total of about 70 exams if there are two sixth-grade classes). Completing these exams in a timely manner is important because until they have been given, nothing else can be accomplished: no health training, disease prevention, or counseling.

If the students do not have a primary care doctor, the health center can provide them with good healthcare for most of their ailments. Many of the students' families do not have access to healthcare, so the families go to the emergency room, where they experience long waiting times before being seen. Charges for emergency departments are much higher than in alternative settings, such as an urgent care clinic or a school health center. Higher charges mean families spend unnecessarily large amounts on their healthcare and/or create huge burdens on national healthcare spending.[2] School health centers offer primary care through an NP for no charge or at greatly reduced rates. Because most of the funding comes through the federal and state governments, costs for great care remain reasonable or low for students who have no health insurance.

Immunizing All School-Aged Children

When Jonnie first arrived at this urban Detroit middle school, she was astounded by the students' lack of healthcare. The immunization rate for the school was between 40 and 50 percent, meaning that 50–60 percent of the students had not been immunized. At that time, there was a tuberculosis epidemic in the area where these children lived, and TB is not something that can be ignored for long. Vaccines do more than produce immunity in those who receive them; they also protect those who come in contact with unvaccinated individuals. Parents who are having difficulty deciding whether to vaccinate their child must consider that vaccinations have saved millions of children (and adults) from the ravages of disease, deformity, disability, and death. Because of vaccines, diseases such as whooping cough, paralytic polio, measles, rubella, meningitis, tuberculosis, chicken pox, and hepatitis B have all but disappeared. Vaccines are critical to the health and well-being of all students.[3]

> Jonnie Hamilton: *I had a student come in for an immunization, which was past due. Now, I never miss an opportunity to give an immunization. This is a transient neighborhood, and sometimes the children won't come to school or they move, so I cannot miss an opportunity to give a vaccine. Vaccinations are so important to the health and well-being of everyone who lives and breathes in a community.*
>
> *I sent a note home, and the mom called back, absolutely irate. "I did not give you permission to give my child a vaccine." I listened carefully and when the parent finally ran out of steam, I spoke. "Do you remember giving me two consents—one for services and one for vaccines? I did attempt to call you, several times, in fact. When I called, I wanted to make you aware that immunizations were past due, and I wanted your permission to give the shot. All of the information about each vaccine was in the pamphlet." Then I asked her, "Is your child okay?"*
>
> *"Yes," the mom answered.*
>
> *Parents want me to call every time I am doing something invasive. But if parents sign the consent form, we can see their children for whatever the symptoms are at the time they present themselves. We have a few parents who won't sign it, but for the most part they do.*

Gaining Parent Trust for a School-Based Health Center

To gain the parents' trust, Jonnie went to every PTA meeting and every open house, where she talked to the parents and they could talk to her. She encouraged the parents to come into the health center so that they could see what she does. She always invited parents to classes on nutrition, hygiene, and asthma, because it is important that parents know exactly what their children are learning. They need to feel comfortable coming to Jonnie for anything.

The students would go home to their parents and say, "*We don't have to go see the doctor anymore. We can go see Nurse Hamilton. She can take care of everything we need.*"

Jonnie has had parents call and ask if there is a doctor's office in the school. She tells them, "*We have a health center in the school. I am a nurse practitioner, and I provide primary care.*" The parents feel good about having the school health center available for themselves and for their school-aged children.

NPs provide treatments for routine illnesses and advise students on how to maintain a healthy lifestyle. They order and interpret diagnostic tests (lab work and x-rays); diagnose and treat chronic conditions such as diabetes, high blood pressure, infections, and injuries; prescribe medications; manage their students' overall care; counsel their students; and help them learn how their actions impact their health and overall well-being. NPs deliver a blend of both nursing and medical care and often serve as the family's primary care provider.[4] However, NPs cannot deliver healthcare all alone; they need support from other school-based NPs and from the medical director for community health at St. John's Providence Health System. NPs and physicians, in collaboration, develop alternative approaches for treating different types of illnesses.

Our job as nurses is to cushion the sorrow and celebrate the joy, every day, while we are just doing our jobs.

—Christine Belle

Developing Patience Under Fire

Jonnie Hamilton: *"A young girl came to me to be tested for chlamydia, and I treated her for the disease. The parent found out and was totally irate. She came storming into my office, yelling, "You can't treat my daughter for this. How do I know that she even has it?" I took the mother to a private room, and she continued to scream at me. She was totally beside herself with anger and frustration, and with her loud voice, others could hear her through the walls. I just sat there and listened and listened and listened some more, always with my full attention. When she was done, I asked her again if she had anything else that she wanted to say. I never interrupt. If you let people vent, eventually they will calm down—but not until they have said all they are going to say.*

I try to be outwardly calm, but inside my head, I am thinking, "Oh, my God." The mom cannot read my face because it is tranquil, but wow! It is difficult to get barraged with so much anger. When the mother was finally done, I said, "In the State of Michigan, when a child reaches the age of thirteen, she can come to the health center without her parent's permission to get help for anything having to do with sexual matters."

"For real?" the mother asked.

"Yes, that is the law." I gave the mother a copy of the law to prove it. "Wouldn't you rather have your child be treated for chlamydia rather than not be treated? Now, tell me what the real problem is."

"The problem is that I did not know my child was sexually active. She did not tell me, but she told you."

"The child was probably afraid of what you might say, or worse yet, what you might do, such as ask her not to see her boyfriend anymore. I would suggest that when you have fully gotten control of your emotions, you talk to her. Give her advice about how to protect herself against chlamydia

and unwanted pregnancies. She will probably continue to have sex, and she might as well be fully informed about the dangers of sex."

Teens and Risky Behavior Involving Alcohol, Drugs, and Early Sex

One-third of all Americans die from their own unhealthy behaviors, and many of these behaviors start during their adolescent years. One major threat to the health of adolescents is their own risky behavior in such things as smoking, abusing alcohol and drugs, and having sex at an early age.[5] When parents direct their children with rewards and threats, the children will look outward for their sense of self. Adopting extrinsic life goals such as wealth, fame, and body image, these adolescents allow their friends and popular culture to dictate what is worth pursuing.

Parents from high-risk neighborhoods often make their teenagers feel less secure about their own safety and more focused on financial success.[6] A follow-up to the Rochester Longitudinal Study involving 140 eighteen-year-olds and their mothers indicated that teenagers and mothers from disadvantaged backgrounds focused on attaining security and a sense of worth from external sources. Mothers living in an environment of uncertainty value conformity more than self-direction and pass those conformist values on to their children. People living in these environments see conformity as necessary to securing a job and often overemphasize the value of money.

Study results showed that mothers in these environments tended to be less nurturing, valuing financial success over self-acceptance and community orientation. Fathers, if they were present at all, tended to ignore their teenagers or provided only minimal fathering care. When directed with rewards, threats, and contingent love, the children experienced distress, and some of them began to lose awareness of their personal needs. Daughters began to engage in early sex. Sons smoked more and began to abuse alcohol, take drugs, and push the limits for health-related risky behaviors.

By contrast, parents who support meaningful relationships and community involvement move their teenagers toward intrinsically motivated goals. Parents who value warmth and autonomy will raise teenagers to also value warmth and autonomy. By acknowledging their teenagers' perspectives and providing them with choices, these parents promote a stronger sense of self-motivated goals and ultimately life goals. Parents who support their teenagers through understanding and appreciation raise teens who are far less likely to engage in early sex, abuse alcohol or drugs, or push the limits for risky teenage behaviors.

If you can give your son or daughter only one gift, let it be enthusiasm.

—Bruce Barton

Motivating Obese Students to Get Active

Jonnie's three main health targets are asthma, hypertension, and obesity. Student hypertension rates are off the charts because the school has a significant number of obese children—30 percent of the students are overweight—and obesity leads to hypertension. "At risk for overweight" refers to children whose body mass index (BMI) for-age is between the 85th and the 95th percentile. In children, "overweight" corresponds to a BMI-for-age greater than the 95th percentile. That is comparable to an adult with a BMI of 30 or more, which is classified as obesity.[7]

For her overweight students, Jonnie has mapped out a mile circuit. If they walk around the school, up the stairs, down the stairs, and back around the school, they will have completed a mile. Jonnie tells them they should do the mile walk at least twice a day, early in the morning and again after lunch. She walks with them to show them the pace, and she outlines where they are to start and finish. However, just showing children what to do doesn't motivate them to complete the mile; for that they need internal motivation. They will not walk the mile if they lack a sense of intention and feel as if they are being pushed to do it. Focusing on intrinsic motivations for healthy living results in greater initial weight loss and better maintenance over a two-year period, according to one study.[8]

Two groups of 528 Hong Kong students[9] participated in a study to examine the difference between the students' self-motivation during a structured physical education lesson led by a teacher and a free-choice period. The students wore a pedometer during a 20-minute structured basketball lesson and a 20-minute free period. The study concluded that the students' self-determination was greater in the free-choice period than in the structured lesson. The adolescents experienced a higher level of self-determined learning that satisfied their psychological needs for autonomy. In other words, Jonnie's overweight students may or may not walk that mile, but "bugging them" will not help. Putting the students into "buddy groups" where they can walk together and socialize may encourage them to walk the mile.

The Importance of Parent Buy-In to Student Health

Jonnie does one-on-one obesity and hypertension education with the students once a month. She also sees them once a month for a weigh-in, to calculate their BMI score, and to measure their blood pressure. Jonnie graphs the results so that the students can see how well they are doing, and maintains an obesity flow sheet so that she knows if they are going up or down. She has had some success, but most of the time the kids stay the same. She has found that if she does not have parent buy-in, the children do not do well.

If the children of parents with weight problems are to do really well at losing weight, their parents must also join the program. When parents cook nutritious food, their
children will eat the same thing. Parents who walk with their children to school instead of driving them establish a pattern. Small

acts count, and they really help with hypertension and obesity. However, if Jonnie does not get the parent buy-in or if a parent is too busy, the end result is generally not successful.

Lifestyle change is an individual choice, and parents often lack the will, the education, the motivation, or the resources to make deep changes in their personal lives. Lifestyle change can have far-ranging effects. Parents have the power to change what they cook, exercise more, and seek healthy choices for their ire family.[10]

Sow an act, and you reap a habit; sow a habit, and you reap a character; sow a character, and you reap a destiny.
—George Dana Boardman

Without parent buy-in, the whole family loses out. All Jonnie can do is educate and hope that all the information she gives parents and their children will sink in. Motivation happens internally, such as when parents and their children cook and eat together. It is not hard to teach the right habits; it's getting students and their parents to follow through that is difficult.

The children have no problem describing a healthy breakfast to Jonnie. They may tell her what they had for dinner and acknowledge that they know it was all-wrong. Children will eat whatever is in the house. When all there is to eat is junk food, children will eat it to survive, but they will not be healthy. That is why parent buy-in is so critical. Over the long term, Jonnie knows that promoting a sense of personal ownership over food consumption is the path to success. That is why she continues to teach her young students about good food and exercise and why both are so important to their health.

When Teaching the Parent Helps the Child

Jonnie Hamilton: *I diagnosed a young man with diabetes and asked him to bring his mom in to see me. When she came in with him, we talked about what kind of foods they usually ate. I asked them both what they knew about diabetes. And I asked the mother, "What do you know about what your child should be eating?" I mentioned that good nutrition would help her son. "If you begin to cook better and he starts to eat better," I said, "he will begin to lose weight and hopefully won't have to go on insulin." The mother shared with me that her husband also has diabetes. Because the father was a diabetic, the mother knew some things about the disease, but because her husband didn't complain, she didn't bother to manage his symptoms with diet, exercise, and proper medication.*

I asked her, "Has your husband ever been to a diabetes class where he could find out about his eating and exercise habits?" I gave her information about the St. John's diabetes class for adults. "Your husband needs to understand about his diagnosis and how he can control his diabetes. He has already had some neuropathy, so we want to make sure that he doesn't have any more symptoms and your son doesn't start developing similar problems."

Weeks later, the father came in to see me. His wife had told him he should talk to me because of my background in diabetes education. He said, "You know, I never would have gone to the class until you told me about my son. I know my wife is going to cook differently and not let me eat this stuff anymore, because she is not going to buy it." The last time I saw the son, he had lost five pounds, which is good but we have a long way to go because he is more than two hundred pounds. This will help the whole family.

Jonnie was practicing the art of good dialogue with these family members to bring out in the open the worrisome thoughts behind the family dynamics. When people feel that their basic needs for autonomy and competence are supported, they respond better to open discussion about care choices. NPs can facilitate discussion about a patient's thoughts and feelings regarding alternative diabetic medications and treatment options and the benefits and drawbacks of each option. NPs who support their patients' self-regulation through proper diet, exercise, and medication use can improve the quality of their patients' lives and their patients' degree of overall life satisfaction.[11]

Treating Asthma with Training and Home Trigger-Proofing

Jonnie gives the teachers in the school a list of the children she thinks would benefit from her classes on nutrition, asthma, hygiene, hand washing, and HIV. The teachers encourage their students to attend Jonnie's classes. The state requires two separate programs, a mental health program and a physical health program. Students from the sixth, seventh, and eighth grade classrooms come for the asthma program. Jonnie teaches them how to use their inhalers both at home and during sports, how to read their peak flow meters, and how to trigger-proof their homes (especially in regard to dust mites).

Asthma is produced when mucus forms in already constricted airways, producing a wheezing sound when the individual breathes out, and when there is prolonged coughing, especially at night or in the early morning.[12] Of the 697 students in Jonnie's school, 85 have been formally diagnosed with asthma. Since the health center opened, Jonnie has offered a six-session asthma training course that teaches students about their medications and their peak flows. Peak flow readings measure lung function so that students can know when they are having a problem.

Jonnie first has students measure their personal best reading when their lungs are well and they can blow. Next, the predicted capacity, which is based on each student's height and weight, is calculated. The zones are red, yellow, and green. Red indicates that a student is having a really big problem; yellow, a problem the student can handle on his or her own; and green, no problem. Jonnie tells the students that if they are feeling fine, they can do their peak flow reading just once a week. If they are not feeling fine, they need to take more than one reading. Asthmatic children need to do a reading before they use their inhalers and again after using them—and then record the findings. Peak flow[13] readings are higher when students are well and lower when their airways are constricted. From changes in recorded values, students and their medical providers can determine lung functionality, severity of asthma symptoms, and treatment options.[14]

> *Asthma research is a lot better and new medicines are always coming out to help young people.*
>
> —Dominique Wilkins

Most of the children know when they are having a problem: their chest hurts and they are wheezing and coughing. But although they know the signs, they don't know what to do next. Jonnie teaches them how to read their inhaler. Most of the time, the children just puff it, and the medication does not get into their lungs and they end up in the emergency department. Jonnie teaches them breathing exercises so that they know how to open their lungs and breathe easier, as well as the proper use of inhalers and nebulizers. Taking a peak flow reading requires the child to take a deep breath, close his or her mouth over the mouthpiece, then blast the air out quickly and record the number. Some of the students have exercise-induced asthma, marked by difficulty breathing and chest tightening when they exert themselves. If they usually start wheezing when running, Jonnie explains to them that they need to use an inhaler before exercise to open their lungs so that they can take part in athletics.

Most children know that dust, mold, cigarette smoke, and roaches will trigger asthma, but they don't know how to trigger-proof their homes. One highly allergic contaminant is house dust, which contains the fecal pellets and skins of dust mites. To control dust mites, the children are taught to put cheesecloth over the heating grates to filter out the mites. They are taught to vacuum their room at least once a day, to wash pillowcases and sheets once a week, to use a nonallergenic pillow, to keep humidity levels below 50 percent, and to use a high-efficiency air filter.[15]

A Student Success Story: Controlling
a Pair of Chronic Illnesses

Jonnie Hamilton: *One student was in our asthma program for three years before he went off to high school. This student's asthma was exacerbated by his sickle-cell anemia. When this student first started attending the program, he was always in a state of crisis with the pain of the sickle-cell anemia and the chronic asthma. The term "sickle-cell crisis" describes several acute conditions in patients with sickle-cell disease. Sickle-cell disease usually occurs in childhood, with about one in five hundred African-American children having the disease. The average life expectancy for a male with the disease is about forty-two years.[16]*

I taught this student how to control his pain by recognizing that blood clots need lots of water. If this student drank water before he started experiencing pain, he could keep the pain from establishing itself. I also taught this student how to meditate by giving him soothing music to listen to when the pain got particularly bad. His mother works in the school, and together we worked hard to provide him with all of the tools he would need to progress to high school.

His mother and I worked on the asthma triggers, using his peak flow parameters, and helped him recognize the signals when he was about to experience an attack. We worked on his exercise, meditation, and water regime. The student graduated [from middle school] *last June and has progressed to high school. I gave the principal at his new high school his Asthma Care Plan and told her that when he says he needs it, he really does. Since he went to high school, he has not experienced another crisis. When he started the program, his grades had fallen to a 1.8 GPA, and in high school his grades have improved to a 2.8. His mother and I feel so proud of this student; he is accomplishing great things.*

Teaching Families to Navigate Detroit's Food Deserts

Many of Detroit's neighborhoods are food deserts, lacking real grocery stores. In the winter, especially, it is difficult to buy fresh foods. Liquor stores hold sway on most corners, and they sell a very limited selection of bread, cereal, milk, and other staples. In these stores fresh fruits and vegetables are nonexistent or moldy. In the summer, markets where families can buy fresh produce from gardeners, farmers, and vendors spring up near schools and in empty lots. But summer goes by fast, and then it is back to purchasing food from gas stations or liquor stores.

When Jonnie talks to parents, she avoids telling them what they should or should not do. She starts off by asking them, especially those who have hypertension and obesity issues, to tell her about their diet and their shopping habits. She uses questions like these to prompt their answers: *"What kinds of foods are available in your local store?" "Do you shop there daily, or is this where you get your basic groceries?" "Do you have transportation?" "How many people are you feeding?"* and *"What is your budget?"*

Once she has the information, she begins to make suggestions, paying careful attention to any feedback she gets. She wants to be sure that it's possible for those she is counseling to do what she is suggesting. She doesn't want to suggest something that she knows they cannot do. For example, if they have transportation once a month, can they go to Costco or Sam's Club? If they cannot buy fresh fruit, can they buy fruit packed in its own juices? Can they buy frozen rather than canned vegetables? What kind of snacks do they usually buy for their children? Can they buy carrot sticks or rice cakes (which will be cheaper than cookies)? Is there something else they could buy in place of cookies that is the same price but a little healthier? Jonnie tell parents that if they buy something unhealthy and do not have anything else in the house, the children will eat whatever is there if they are hungry.

Water and juice are each cheaper than soda pop. Flavored juices can be very expensive; for example, a ten-pack of Capri Sun costs $3, or 30¢ a packet. Many people drink bottled water because they do not like the taste of their local water or question its safety. At a dollar or more a bottle, though, bottled water is both overpriced and, in all reality, not really any better than the local tap water. The parents might say, *"I don't like tap water."* Jonnie tells them to boil it, strain it through cheesecloth, and put it in the refrigerator. The cost of a pitcher and cheesecloth, both of which can be purchased for a dollar, is a much better bargain than bottled water.

Jonnie hands out brochures about nutritious foods to the parents so that they know what to buy. She encourages parents to watch the papers for sales. She reminds them that they do not have to buy brand names, like Cheerios. Instead, they should compare Cheerios to the grocery-store brand; not only will the unbranded cereal be cheaper, but the package will be bigger. The grocery store will also have sales on bread, often ten loaves for $10. Jonnie encourages them to buy the wheat bread; it provides better nutrition for them and their children. Jonnie's brochures contain great tips on how to select healthy snacks that can keep children's energy levels high and minds alert, and provide the vitamins and nutrients children's growing bodies need.

Listening Without Judging and Teaching Options for Healthy Living

As a nurse practitioner, Jonnie does not share her personal beliefs or values with parents or students unless they ask her what she thinks. She refrains from telling them what they should do because she found early in her career that this did not work. Parents and students have their own values, and change needs to happen from the inside out. Jonnie strives to give parents and students enough options so that they can make choices about their lifestyle.

Jonnie listens to parents and students without judgment. Her aim is to help families make good choices about their lives. She empowers them by helping them shift their beliefs about their own health. The more they know, the better they can deal with the health system and the more they can advocate for themselves. So,

Jonnie gives them as much oral and written information as possible. She tells them that if they do not understand what the doctors are saying, to just ask them to explain.

For example, if a doctor tells someone that their cholesterol is 190 and then says nothing else, they will not know what to do or how to control it. Jonnie explains that a normal cholesterol benchmark is below 150 for children and below 200 for adults, and that the doctor can explain ways to control high cholesterol. Jonnie feels confident that by providing simple advice like this, she can change how parents interact with physicians and help them get their questions answered.

Measuring Results with GPA Scores and School Attendance

Jonnie Hamilton's work has produced some measurable results: fewer missed days of school, higher GPA scores, and fewer emergency room visits among the students at her school. This is especially true for her asthma students. At the start of each asthma program, the school gives student participants a pretest and a posttest and then compares students' GPAs before and after they complete the class. GPA scores are 2–3 points higher for each student in the "deep breath" program. The number of days absent from school before and after the class has decreased by 2–3 days, and the number of emergency room visits has decreased to 0–1 for each student. The asthma students have gradually gained ground and are successfully transitioning from middle to high school without skipping a beat.

Obesity results are slowly improving as well. One investigation of a link between obesity and school performance suggests that obese children and adolescents miss more school days than their thinner cohorts and experience gaps in knowledge, especially when taking tests.[17] A solution is to require physical education and to push for reforms in eating behaviors, such as eating more fruits and vegetables and not purchasing foods high in fat, sodium, or added sugars.[18] Ever so slowly, GPA scores at Jonnie's school are improving, and students are better able to transition from middle school to high school with improved grades and a happier outlook on life.

Jonnie's hope is that everyone who needs healthcare will receive it in a timely manner and that parents and students should be able to see a primary care doctor. Good preventive care can save everyone a lot of money, as can teaching people about exercise and good nutrition from the start. Asthma, obesity, and diabetes are on the rise, so it is important that children get care early and often.

More about Jonnie Hamilton

I started out as a diploma nurse, and my first job as a new grad was working the midnight shift at Mt. Carmel Mercy Hospital in Detroit, Michigan. At that time, you did everything as a brand-new grad, and my feet were really put to the fire. I learned more there than I ever would have somewhere else. I can tell you that the licensed practical nurses (LPNs) working there saved me many a day. Even though they didn't have the degree, they knew more than I did because they had been working there longer and just knew what to do. I had the degree but did not know everything.

Later, the LPNs told me that they appreciated my asking them what to do. I had the degree, but they had the practical knowledge. Actually, all five of the LPNs who worked at Mt. Carmel then are now registered nurses (RNs). I told them, "There is no reason that you should hold yourself back. You know more than most. Now just get the degree and learn to apply that knowledge." They later told me that it was the best information they had received.

I got my nurse practitioner (NP) degree from the University of Michigan in Ann Arbor, when it was a two-year certificate program, not a master's program. (After 1985 it became a master's program.) The doctors at the University of Michigan Health Service were all NP friendly, so they were great to work with, and we learned a lot. When Sinai-Grace Hospital in Detroit came, I stayed in the same building and kept practicing. Then I moved to the Detroit Medical Center (DMC), where I worked for five years before taking on my current role as the nurse practitioner for this school-based health center.

How Ms. Hamilton Uses Her Leadership Skills to Empower Students and Families Regarding Their Health

In the seventeen years that Jonnie has been the director of the Napoleon Jordan Center for HealthCare at Marcus Garvey Academy in Detroit, she has done so many things for her students and their families. She can look back and measure the progress she has made at her school health center. Jonnie has:

- Conducted school health exams until every last child has been immunized and provided with a thorough school physical.

- Gained the trust of parents by inviting them to participate in classes, visit the school health center, and realize that care is available for themselves and their school-aged children.

- Served as the primary care provider for students and their families by focusing on health promotion, disease prevention, health education, and counseling.

- Learned patience, when to listen and practice good dialogue, and when to step in with health education tips.

- Understood that overweight students (and their parents) need to develop personal ownership over their food consumption and exercise.

- Sent one diabetic student's father to a diabetes class offered at St. John's Providence, and now the family eats better and both father and son control their diabetes.

- Provided a six-week training course that teaches students how to use their nebulizers, trigger-proof their homes against allergens, and take the proper medications.

- Taught families to navigate Detroit's food deserts by engaging in a dialogue about diet and shopping habits and by providing brochures describing good, nutritious foods.

- Empowered parents and students to shift their beliefs about their own health and become advocates for wise lifestyle choices.

- Seen the results of her work in higher GPA scores, fewer days absent from school, and fewer emergency room visits.

Conclusion

School-based health centers can play an important role in ensuring that students and their families can experience good primary healthcare. Staff at these centers can treat illnesses and help students and families maintain a healthy lifestyle. NPs can order diagnostic tests; diagnose and treat chronic conditions such as diabetes, high blood pressure, and asthma; prescribe medications; and manage each student's overall care. They can deliver high-quality, personalized health education and counseling while providing a blend of nursing and medical care that can lower healthcare costs for students and their families.

School based health centers play an important part in maintaining a healthy living style for all families and students. Nursing schools need to pay more attention to offering nurse practitioners for schools across the country. Often the school centers operate as partners with community health centers, hospitals and the health department with ongoing care provided between the organizations. Currently there are nearly 2,000 school health centers across the country. The Affordable Care Act provides a total of $200 million through 2013 to support capital grants to improve services at these centers and $95 million was awarded to 278 schools, enabling them to serve an additional 440,000 patients. With these funds, schools can modernize, build new facilities and purchase much needed equipment to increase access for their students and families.[19]

Actions for Nurse Practitioners

Question for Reflection

Reaching out to patients is critical to forming a bond with them. What can you do to understand your patients and validate your assumptions about what they may be thinking or feeling? How can you convey that understanding to your patients without appearing to be disingenuous or pandering?

Reaching Out

- Go into the community, and validate your data with the people you seek to serve. Learn to sell yourself and how you plan to conduct their care.
- Share quality statistics to support your areas of treatment, and explain how you plan to treat the condition, be it a chronic problem, the flu, or something else.

Example:

To gain the trust of patients in the community, you need to go out into the community and sell your services. Most nurses are extremely uncomfortable with this aspect of care, but it is necessary. Let your patients know what you are doing, and broadcast the quality of what you do. Have the statistics to back up your claims and best-practice evidence to prove you know about their illness.

Listening to Patients

- Listen carefully to understand the meaning behind the words. Often what remains unsaid reveals what is really going on.
- Give honest and direct answers to patient questions.

Example:

You can learn so much by listening to your patients. If you listen hard enough, patients will give you a clue about what is going on. Ask directed questions that probe deeper and deeper. Nurse practitioners have that special knack for asking questions that reveal "hidden" patient concerns. Often the "real" issue has nothing to do with the problem the patient originally came in to discuss.

Training Asthma Students

- Teach students about how dust, mold, cigarette smoke, and roaches can trigger asthma, and help them learn strategies for trigger-proofing their homes.
- Instruct students in when and how to use their medications and how to take peak flow readings, which measure lung function, so that they will know when they are having a problem.

Example:

Build trust with your students by teaching them how to reduce allergens in their homes by putting cheesecloth over the heating vents to keep out dust, mold, and dust mites. Explain to asthmatic patients that they need to do a reading before they use their inhalers and again after using them— and then record the findings. Patients will often give you clues about their home situation if you pay attention.

Empowering Others

- Develop relationships with patients so that they understand that you are invested in their care.
- Educate patients by providing them with options for their care. Help them make the right decisions about themselves and how they want to be treated.

Example:

Bring good data to the table, and encourage people to use it to make educated decisions about their healthcare. Consider handing out brochures that explain treatment options for asthma, hypertension, obesity, and diabetes; help patients understand their options. Teach patients to ask probing questions about their own health. Never assume that you know it all.

Motivating Patients

- Help patients develop commitment to and personal ownership of their goals, especially around healthy behavior.
- When you give patients the responsibility to set their own goals, respect the goals they set.

Example:

Patients know themselves. Respect their autonomy in setting their own goals so that they will be more likely to sustain the behaviors that will support their long-term health and well-being. People who feel supported can more readily embrace a healthier lifestyle and a better quality of life. Advice giving, lecturing, and coercion don't move patients toward a healthier way of living.

CHAPTER SEVEN

The Acute Care Nurse Practitioner: Building Positive Relationships Between Hospital and Faculty and with Physicians

The demand for acute care nurse practitioners (ACNPs) across hospitals, emergency rooms, specialty clinics, and especially in the intensive care unit (ICU) is on the rise as seniors live longer because of advances in medical care. There are now more than 3,500 advanced practice nurses who have been certified as ACNPs, and that number is continually expanding.[1] The Leapfrog Group has a commitment to inform patients about hospital safety and promote full disclosure of hospital performance information.[2] One of the group's recommendations is a mandate that critical care must be available at the patient's bedside within five minutes. Residents cannot always be present because of work-hour restrictions, and physicians cannot keep up with the increasing need for critical care services.

In the ICU setting, ACNPs can provide quality care, help decrease length of hospital stay, improve patient and family satisfaction, increase communication among medical team members, and advance overall patient care. In addition, they can provide patients, their families, and staff with education, consultation, and care coordination throughout the hospital stay.[3] ACNPs also assist in the teaching of residents (who often rotate through the ICU for only a month) and provide instruction on the many protocols used in the ICU.

Teaching hospitals also offer ACNPs with excellent opportunities to practice with and learn from surgeons of all types.[4] Generally affiliated with a university medical school, teaching hospitals have a commitment to conduct research, providing experimental and innovative services to push the boundaries of medicine. Teaching hospitals have long been considered places of excellence where residents, student nurses, and other health professionals can gather experience as they encounter complicated cases and then apply their learning to other patients.

One ACNP's Many Achievements

Laurie Hartman practiced in many nursing roles until she found what some might call her dream job. As an ACNP and a DNP, she serves as both the Director of Advanced Practice Nursing at the University of Michigan Hospital System (UMHS) and as Clinical Assistant Professor at the U-M School of Nursing (SON). Since her appointment to these positions in July 2010, Laurie has worked to build understanding of professional nurse practitioner (NP) roles, foster connections, and uphold practice standards.[5] For example, she has advocated for an NP orientation program, fostered connections between the nursing school and the hospital, and encouraged her advanced practice nurses (APNs) to keep up-to-date on regulations at the national and state levels and to keep residents current on ICU protocols.

As both a professor and a clinical director, Laurie exercises significant influence in connecting the U-M SON and the UMHS and in building relationships between the hospital's NP staff and the SON faculty. However, she was initially surprised at the disconnect that she identified between the hospital NPs and the nursing faculty. Laurie's goal, which she is working with the SON's dean to achieve, is to build synergistic relationships between the SON and the UMHS, to increase collaboration between the entities.

Laurie values the profession of nursing and focuses efforts on building support within the hospital for the profession and for advanced education for nurses. With both words and deeds, Laurie encourages her staff and coworkers by modeling what she expects others to do. She has established an orientation process within the

UMHS, and she helps link students in the SON's ACNP program with faculty members to strengthen bonds between the students and their ACNP mentors. She shows the student nurses that no one should pass by a patient's call light without stopping and checking. Drawing on her own clinical experiences, including her mistakes, she encourages students to learn and grow from her examples. She advocates for NP students by modeling leadership and oversees the NP privileging process, thereby reinforcing NP professional practice standards.

Laurie also works to address and strengthen hiring practices for NPs. Shortly after assuming her leadership post; she sought increased recognition for all APNs. Historically, there have been some hiring challenges in some departments because UMHS APNs work under a union contract and physician assistants (PAs) do not. In an effort to understand system barriers and clarify UMHS regulations, Laurie collaborated with human resources and union leadership to change job-posting classifications so that APNs would be eligible to apply for open NP and PA positions in the hospital.

Moving the Needle to Establish a
Shared Governance Model

Since APNs at the UMHS function in a decentralized structure, one of Laurie's first endeavors was to create a governance model that aligned with the nursing governance model of the UMHS. The model called for involvement, open communication, and collaboration across APNs in all departments. Laurie understands the transformational power of having 400 APNs meet to develop and take ownership of a shared-governance and shared-leadership structure. Her vision of practice is inspirational, and she uses as her operative motto, *"Together we mean something."*[6]

Laurie imparts her fervent belief in APN power to all 400 APNs across all departments. She challenges APNs to dream big about the future possibilities of healthcare and their place in it. Changing to a shared-governance model requires shifts in perception of what quality healthcare really means.[7] Shared governance demands collaborative relationships between physicians and APNs, improves quality of care, increases staff confidence, facilitates development of skills, increases accountability, and encourages open sharing of information. Shared governance should be a fluid process, requiring ongoing evaluation of what works and what needs re-evaluation.

To Laurie, transforming healthcare also means transforming the culture of advanced practice nursing to one of shared sacrifice and ongoing commitment. It means questioning the "rules for engagement" and sharing success stories from other services. It means understanding that one size does not fit all departments and that each department needs to establish its own culture. It means that all APNs need to be valued, respected, protected by their physician and their nurse manager, and supported in developing professional acumen.[8] A shared governance model cannot be developed in six months; it requires extensive leadership, consideration, and active planning. Governance plans are critical for developing ongoing collaboration between healthcare providers, improving quality of care, increasing communication, and fostering trust.

Enhancing Leadership Abilities through Interpersonal Skills

Though Laurie manages all 400 APNs, she maintains a special relationship with Melissa Baldwin and Erin Lindstrom, her two ACNPs working in the ICU. They focus on the condition of each patient, along with the effects of illness on the lives of patients and their families. ACNPs often work as go-betweens with regard to communication between the physician and the patient, their families, and other members of the patient's healthcare team. Two-thirds of ACNPs work in a hospital inpatient setting, and the other third work in the ICU. Because Laurie started her career in the ICU, she keeps close watch on these two ACNPs; in her heart she will always maintain an affiliation with severely ill patients.

Laurie inspires confidence by how she speaks and how she

influences others. She knows that to be a good leader, she needs the support of her APNs, the physicians, and, most important, her superiors. Laurie understands the social psychology of power and uses the principles of power to enhance her interpersonal interactions.[9] For example, psychologist Carl Rogers defines empathy as *"entering the private perceptual world of the other and becoming thoroughly at home in it. It involves being sensitive, moment to moment, to the changing felt meanings which flow in this other person."*[10] Laurie fosters these felt meanings.

Laurie consistently works to improve her listening skills and encourages her staff, Melissa and Erin, to do the same. Laurie applauds Erin's mastery of good listening and ability to summarize the core messages of a communication. Rather than simply telling those she is teaching what to do, Erin instead opens a dialogue about various procedures and their impacts on the patient. Laurie gives this example:

> Laurie Hartman: *When Erin talks to a resident, she listens to his or her ideas and guides him or her to a plan. For example, when a resident asks her what the plan is for the day, Erin might respond: "For a post-op heart-bypass patient, what do you think the plan should be? Based on the guidelines that you know, what do you think should be done?"*
>
> *Sometimes it would be easier just to tell the questioner the answer, but Erin wants the resident to think about the plan and any follow-up actions. Sometimes certain surgeons want things done one way and other surgeons want them done another way. Erin might ask the resident to consider the differences between processes for a mitral valve and a tricuspid valve. It is all about opening a dialogue about why we do what we do. Sometimes there is no "right" or "wrong" way to get to the end point. If an approach is not detrimental to the patient, then it is okay.*

Increasing Collaboration across Departments

Laurie continuously watches for opportunities to increase collaboration between floors, departments, and units. She encourages her APNs to take on new roles and pushes them to address difficult issues. By encouraging her APNs to grow and expand their limits, she gives them permission to challenge established boundaries, identify "stretch" goals, and achieve organizational goals. She works to eliminate such statements as *"We never do it that way"* or *"That won't work."* She empathizes with her team's perspective while challenging them to explore alternative methods for change.

For example, there were issues at hand-off when patients were transferred from the ICU to the step-down unit. Laurie describes how her ACNP handled the situation:

Laurie Hartman: *Melissa stepped in and helped the step-down unit understand how their processes impacted the ICU and how the ICU handled and transferred patients to the step-down unit. She drew on her leadership qualities, such as passion for her work, and helped both teams think about their own processes and how they could change them so that the transition would run smoothly.*

Together, the two teams [the ICU and the step-down unit] generated new processes based on consensus. They asked themselves: "What does the ICU consider to be necessary in taking a patient to the step-down unit?" "What does the step-down unit need to consider when receiving a patient who is being transferred from the ICU?" Each department, the ICU and the step-down unit, walked the other through all of the steps it felt were needed. Until each department understood what the other department faced, moving forward was impossible. Finally, when each department understood the other's viewpoint, they could agree on the processes necessary to move the patient between the different units.

Melissa brought her infectious enthusiasm to bear to push the departments to acknowledge and encourage all ideas. By openly and enthusiastically recognizing the "goodness" in all ideas, she got people to open up and share. Ideas can come from the most unlikely places, and Melissa encouraged the departments to think creatively. She reminded the nurses that a smooth path does not always lead to success. Tough choices require that people take risks and push themselves to go above and beyond what they think is possible.

Process improvements can enhance working structures and systems. Increases in staff skills can improve quality of care, create a positive culture, and provide a proactive learning environment. Moving a patient from one floor to another requires carefully thinking through all of the steps necessary to make it right. What needs to happen first? How can the process steps be improved? What happens at the point of transfer? It is not easy to move patients, and even small changes can have a major impact on overall patient care. Process changes enhance clinical effectiveness and ensure that practices are based on the best possible evidence.[11]

Ever-Changing Team Dynamics and True Listening Skills

One of the biggest challenges to any nursing team, particularly one in a teaching hospital, is the ever-changing composition of the larger healthcare team of which they are a part. Change has become a constant. While the patient is hospitalized in the ICU, he or she is assigned to the care of a surgeon, who performs the operative procedures he or she needs. A medical team that includes an attending physician,[12] a staff physician who has completed residency and practices in a clinic or hospital, handles the day-to-day care of the patient while the surgeon is operating on other patients.

Then there are groups of residents, fellows, and interns who work under the oversight of an intensivist (an anesthesiologist with critical care training who works in the ICU)[13] to provide the patient's day-to-day care. Although the surgeons remain the same, every week there is a new attending physician and a new intensivist, and every month the residents and interns change. Melissa and Erin need to understand each new attending's communication style and clinical management practices—not an easy task. The ACNP team has to navigate all of those challenges and collaborate with the bedside nursing staff and with the surgeon or attending, who periodically participates in decisions about the patient's care plan.

The surgeon will develop the patient plan of care, and then the ACNP team will take over from there. Melissa and Erin perform the critical task of relaying clinical changes in the patient's condition to other members of the team and working through how the staff will coordinate the patient's care. There is minimal time for questions when getting the surgeon's consensus or attempting to steer the patient's care in a different direction. In addition, Melissa and Erin need to be up-to-date on evolving national and local standards of care. Because residents rotate constantly, many are not familiar with the ICU protocols. The ACNPs need to provide the necessary continuity, making sure that all targets are hit and the documentation required for reimbursement is completed.

How do APNs learn to listen to everything that is happening around them while maintaining an outward calm? They learn to take a deep interest in what others say. They watch closely for body language and facial expressions that often convey more information than words can. They work hard to take varying points of view and connect them together into summary points that convey points of view from all sides.[14] Everybody loves to be asked for his or her opinion. Being asked makes people feel involved in the dialogue and elicits valuable information from them. APNs learn to work with varied physician personality types and to switch between firm and nice approaches as needed. Their ability to truly listen to multiple team members helps bridge differences of opinion into a coherent approach.

Happiness is a conscious choice, not an automatic response.
—Mildred Barthel

In one study of 65 community nurses, working in 13 teams, members of each team recorded their moods and the number of hassles they had with their teammates daily. The results displayed an association between the nurses' daily moods and the collective moods of the rest of their team. The older the nurse, the greater the correlation, particularly if the nurse perceived the working climate to be positive, experienced fewer hassles with teammates, and was committed to the team.[15] In other words, a nurse can lift the climate of the room or take it down. Upholding standards of care remains critical, but a positive attitude can positively affect an extended team.

Influences on Physician-Patient Communication and Interaction

Laurie Hartman: *To give the physicians credit, they are also working on their communication skills. I have seen big changes in how they are relating to people and how they express themselves. The practice of medicine is based on highly personal interactions between surgeons and patients. The more surgeons can elicit the worries and fears of their patients, the more they can connect with them on an emotional level.*

In one study, surgeons rated their liking for some patients higher than for others. The better the physical and emotional health of the patient, the more the surgeons responded favorably to them. Patients with more education and higher incomes scored significantly higher on the "like" scale than less well educated, lower income, and more vulnerable patients. Sick patients reduce surgeon satisfaction. Happier surgeons, those who are satisfied with their careers, have more emotional energy to give to their patients. Surgeons under a great deal of stress may be less flexible in personal relationships with patients.[16] In general, surgeons need be mindful of their emotional well-being and of any inappropriate biases they may have toward their patients, especially if the patients are very sick and/or very poor. Positive relationships increase patient trust; negative interactions destroy it.

Even though surgeons may feel good about their patient, in the operating room they can be very intense, especially when operating on a patient's heart. Even when the cardiac surgeon executes flawlessly, sometimes the outcome is not positive. After working on an intricate and difficult surgery for twelve hours, the surgeon must hand over control of the patient's care to the ICU team. The surgeon cannot necessarily predict what will happen to the patient when he or she leaves to go home. Some patients may not make it through the night, no matter how good the care they receive.

How Proactive Patient Care Builds Trust

Caring theory demonstrates that when nurses care about their patients, they react more quickly to their patients' needs.[17] Identifying and responding to the patient's needs without being asked sends a powerful message—a message that the nurse really cares. When a nurse goes into a patient's room, introduces herself, explains her role, calls the patient by his or her preferred name, and sits with the patient and the family for five minutes, the patient begins to trust the nurse. Patients and their families gain a sense of control and feel they can actively participate in the care.[18] Of all the skills nurses need to develop, listening is the most critical because it helps to build the trust that is necessary for the staff to initiate healthcare procedures.

One person caring about another represents life's greatest value.

—Jim Rohn

Time spent sitting by the bedside actively listening to problems, feelings, and concerns builds trust. Touching an arm to show support builds trust. Expressing concern for the family and making sure that they know the plan builds trust. Encouraging patients to take active control over their bodies and their environment builds trust. Good relationships are based on the patient's and family's faith that the healthcare staff will take excellent care of the patient and provide him or her with the best services possible.

Laurie Hartman describes how Melissa and Erin build trust with their ICU patients:

Laurie Hartman: *Every morning, Melissa goes into each patient's room and introduces herself: "Hi, I'm Melissa, and I am your nurse practitioner." She asks patients how they are feeling and how their night was. Then she tells them, "Here is what I am thinking for today. The surgeon will be around shortly. You will see a whole group of people doing rounds; please ask any questions you want during rounds. If you have any concerns, please let me know."*

Erin and Melissa try hard to help families understand what is going on in the middle of the controlled chaos that is the ICU. They work hard at establishing good relationships, but patients and their families often become confused over all the attention they are receiving, asking, "Why are all of these people working with me?" Erin and Melissa tell them: "You may hear a lot of words that you do not understand, confusing words that hold little or no meaning. We will come back and explain what all the medical terms mean and how you can determine their significance."

Melissa or Erin explains to the patient or a family member what will happen during grand rounds. [Grand rounds, which involve presenting each patient's medical problem and treatment to doctors, residents, and medical students, are an important teaching tool.][19] *They want the family to ask questions, especially if the patient feels any pain or needs anything.* [The UMHS went from never having patients and family members ask questions during rounds to almost always inviting them to join in.]

The architecture of the small, cramped ICU room makes it difficult for the attending physician, surgeon, intensivist, and resident all to fit around the bed, especially with the wires and other equipment in the room. Therefore, after everyone has left, Melissa or Erin circles back and shares the plan for the day, which may involve taking the patient off some of the lines, getting him or her up and moving and walking, or having the patient stay in bed and just be still.

The ACNPs form a bridge between the surgeons and the family, across which clinical information about what is going on and what will happen next can be conveyed. ACNPs form the strategic bond that cements good relationships between all parties, working collectively for the health of the patient and encouraging the patient to take active control of his or her well-being. ACNPs can sit with a patient to give family members and friends' time to walk through the gardens, sit in the cafeteria, and get away from the cramped ICU room. Having the chance to walk, breathe, eat, and drink can make returning to the room bearable.

Studies suggest how important it is to respond to a patient's request quickly. The more physicians, residents, nurses, and support staff communicate directly with the patient, the higher the patient satisfaction scores. When all members of the interdisciplinary team listen, communicate, and coordinate care, clinical outcomes improve and cost savings are seen. Satisfied patients return to the facility for future care and recommend the facility to friends and relatives, increasing market share and revenues.

Helping Patients Cope with Anxiety

Patients in the ICU environment generally are anxious, even those with a favorable prognosis. Uncertainty about one's illness, particularly a recurring illness, can be emotionally crippling. Patients who use medical search engines to research their illness often exhibit heightened fears and emotional distress. Many ICU patients are facing the need to learn to live with the new reality of their disease and must learn new coping skills.

Erin Lindstrom has an ICU patient who needs surgery but must wait for more than a week until the surgeon, who has multiple competing demands on his time, can attend to her. Meanwhile, both the patient and her husband are on the edge emotionally. Erin makes it a point to update both of them at least four times a day; even the tiniest report helps keep their emotions in check. Erin understands their nervousness; anxiety can become more pronounced when coupled with uncertainty. Although there is nothing Erin can do to alleviate the fears of a patient facing an intricate and complex surgery, she practices the art of emotional positivity. With every piece of information, no matter how small, that Erin provides, the patient feels better. Anything that helps people feel good—laughter or a well-timed joke, for example—improves work quality and care quality. When the patient feels better, the ACNP feels better, and anxiety goes down.

Understanding What to Share with Patients and Their Families

From the physician's perspective, balancing the patient's medical care needs with the family's needs for information can be a challenge. The physician might convey information about a patient's prognosis to a resident that he or she might not tell a family member. Residents focus primarily on the disease and its treatment: *"What do I need to do? What are the plans?"* The residents do the hands-on physical care and need assurance that they are doing the right thing. Finding a cure forms the medical focus at UMHS.

Laurie Hartman: *We constantly try to balance what can be shared and at what level of detail. We want to balance the teaching and the sharing in equal portions. Rotating residents need the basics of handling seriously ill patients in the ICU, listening to the reasons behind each surgical decision, and maintaining patient kindness. Surgical residents need to learn about being clinically excellent without compromising patient care. Patients and families need honest information about the prognosis of the disease and how to choose different options of care.*

Many ICU patients are anxious about their health, especially when faced with an illness that can recur. To handle these medical anomalies, ACNPs assess their patients, plan and implement the steps for their care, and communicate and coordinate the care plan. They provide a vital presence on the unit, serving as liaisons between all the disciplines and ensuring quality care. They provide a vital communication link between the healthcare team and the patient. Some ACNPs follow patients into their homes or long-term care facilities to ensure a successful transition after discharge.

The Night Life of an ACNP

Night work can be crazy at times. In the UMHS ICU, interns, residents, and one ACNP manage twenty-four patients and a number of fresh post-ops, all of whom require constant surveillance. Monitors are everywhere: on the walls and hanging from the ceilings. Erin and Melissa use their organizational and collaborative skills to care for the fresh post-ops and to check on patients in their rooms. Sometimes the work requires them to sit with patients and talk about how they are coping with their illness. At other times, when patients are too sick to talk, caring might mean just a simple touch on the hand or arm. Neither the intensivist nor the fellow stays with patients' overnight, unless the ACNP team needs them to, such as in an emergency situation.

There is a bone deep security that goes with the brush of a human hand, a silent, reflex-level affirmation that someone is near, that someone cares.

—Jim Butcher, *White Night*

In a code situation, Erin or Melissa will be on the phone with the attending physician and the intensivist while at the same time running the code.

> Laurie Hartman: *During a code, we need to stay calm, organized, and on top of the situation. The challenge can be exhilarating, and we do everything to handle the code. It is not our job to fix everything, but it is our job to notice a problem and get the proper people in here to help out.*

The medical team, including the surgeon, the intensivist, and the surgical residents, comment on the tremendous amount of respect they have for what the ACNPs can do. They trust them to recognize and respond to emergencies; otherwise, the physicians would not be able to leave the hospital. The ACNPs work effectively with many different personalities and respond to many different demands. They interact with medical professionals and patients and their families all day long and collaborate between all of the different needs. Erin and Melissa rely on each other a lot, pitching in and helping each other out. Each has developed strong relationships with the physicians, who rely on the ACNPs to do the right thing by their patients and the families, especially at night.

A Physician Advocate for Mid-level Providers

Dr. Richard Prager is a professor of surgery, the division head of adult cardiac surgery, and the director and clinical lead for the Cardiovascular Center. Because of his positive experiences working with PAs and NPs, Dr. Prager has become a strong advocate for mid-level providers. He has persuaded physicians who preferred to work only with PAs or only with NPs to understand both roles and the specific qualifications of each. He teaches colleagues to understand advanced-practice functions, by explaining how the distinct skill sets of these roles can improve patient care.

PAs conduct physical exams, diagnose and treat illnesses, order and interpret tests, counsel on preventive healthcare, assist in surgery, give medical orders, and write prescriptions.[20] APNs, including certified nurse practitioners, clinical nurse specialists, certified nurse anesthetists, and certified nurse midwives, provide care for patients across a wide variety of healthcare settings. They practice across the country in hospitals, community clinics, schools, retail organizations, and universities, as well as internationally. APNs have highly positive results on patient follow-up; consultation; satisfaction; and screenings, assessments, and counseling.

When Laurie Hartman returned to the UMHS from the University of Pittsburgh Medical Center in 2001, she joined forces with Dr. Prager. The two have worked together to evolve mid-level practice for more than a decade. Laurie offers a perspective rooted in her experiences directing 400 APNs and leading the practice of NP care across the hospital. Dr. Prager offers his seasoned insights as a cardiac surgeon and clinical lead for the Cardiovascular Center. They work together quite well.

Dr. Prager: *I came from an environment where we covered the entire ICU with one critical care intensivist and the rest PAs. In academic settings, the focus is on educating and training physicians and understanding how PAs and NPs can be your colleagues. Being able to trust that the NP or PA will support physicians in their work goes a long way to creating effective and collaborative relationships.*

I see absolutely no challenges and zero issues in having a team concept where people from different backgrounds all work together to deliver good cardiac care. In an institution like this, I would be disappointed if there was not a full integration of all these people into one team, where everyone works together in a collaborative fashion. Everyone has unique talents to bring to the care of our patients.

Resident-Hour Limits and Care Service Changes

When Dr. Prager arrived at University of Michigan's Cardiovascular Center, his two main goals were caring for patients and educating residents.

Dr. Prager: *When I got here, the residents slept here and were on call until they dropped. A well-appointed care team was not really necessary; we did everything for the patients. Then residents reduced their hours to the eighty-hour workweek, and we could no longer keep them working so hard. We had to make room for more robust care services and bring in mid-level providers. This forced institutions like the University of Michigan Hospital System into recognizing simple facts about hiring PAs and NPs and fitting them into the treatment plans.*

Increasing Training Opportunities for All

Dr. Prager: *With nursing schools, medical schools, and PAs wanting master's degrees, the competition for training opportunities abounds. I personally believe we should have a PA school; PAs' training is historically different, with completely different platforms. We limit ourself as an institution without having more access to PAs. This concerns me for the future.*

The nursing schools want to educate advanced practice nurses in clinical care or in Doctor of Nurse Practitioner programs, thus setting up competition with medical students and residents. Frankly, with so much work to do, so what if there is competition? With so many patients for us to see and too little time to see them, we cannot be bothered with turf battles over who does what and to whom.

Doing More with Less

Dr. Prager: *Last year, we worked on nine percent more heart patients and did not change our manpower. It was a huge accomplishment. We broke ourselves a little bit, but just intermittently. Some of the patients were dissatisfied, and with them, we spent time actively listening to descriptions of their problems and concerns. Ultimately, we recognized what had happened and began to work on fixes.*

As for productivity, we need to start simple and ask, how much can one person accomplish in twelve hours? Today, we had no resident in the OR and did four heart surgeries. We did that with three PAs, one being on winter break and the other being out with a cut finger. Everybody just stepped up. As a matter of professionalism, we expect that everyone will come through—and they do what is needed.

One Nurse's Leadership Accomplishments

Laurie Hartman has done so much to promote advanced practice nursing as the Director of Advanced Practice Nursing at the UMHS and Clinical Assistant Professor at the U-M SON.

- Laurie has fostered linkages between the hospital APNs and SON faculty members by strengthening the connections between the two organizations.

- Laurie has established an orientation process within the UMHS, and helps link students in the SON's ACNP program with faculty members to strengthen bonds between the students and their ACNP mentors.

- From a decentralized structure, Laurie created a governance model that aligned 400 APNs across all hospital departments and created involvement, open communication, and collaboration and shared leadership.

- She collaborated with human resources and union leadership to change job-posting classifications so that APNs would be eligible to apply for open NP and PA positions in the hospital.

- Laurie encourages process improvements to heighten quality of care, especially when patient transitions from one department to another require detailed plans and a coordinated effort.

- Laurie encourages APNs to keep up-to-date on regulations at the national and state levels and to keep residents current on ICU protocols.

- Laurie advances a caring process that builds patient and family trust by listening to their needs and furthering their sense of control.

- Laurie insists that APNs share the plan of care with each ICU patient and family, to bridge what is happening clinically and what will happen next.

- She also calls for balancing patients' medical care needs with the needs of their families and balancing teaching and sharing.

Conclusion

Currently there are 5,000 ACNPs working in hospitals across the United States.[21] The primary functions of those ACNPs are to assess patient conditions, implement medical management plans, coordinate plans of care, and act as a liaison with other members of the healthcare team to provide evidence-based, quality care. ACNPs collaborate closely with physicians and other members of the healthcare team in generating plans of care. In addition, many ACNPs plan staff educational activities, participate on hospital committees and in research activities, and work with university-based nursing schools.

ACNPs provide care across a wide variety of hospital settings, including inpatient settings, hospital to clinic, emergency departments, intensive care units, specialty laboratories, and acute and subacute care wards. ACNPs teach patients and their families how to work with residents, intensivists, and surgeons to guarantee that they will receive the very best of care related to acute surgical difficulties, care-plan continuity, and patient safety concerns. The Leapfrog Group reports that one benefit of ACNP coverage in the ICU is that an ACNP can be by a critically ill patient's side within five minutes. In a literature review, Margaret Fry[22] demonstrated that ACNPs improved patient flow and clinical outcomes by reducing patient complications and morbidity and mortality rates. Studies have also demonstrated positive financial outcomes related to reduced ICU length of stay, hospital length of stay, and re-admission rates.

Actions for Nurse Practitioners

Question for Reflection

How do successful leaders create an environment of enthusiasm and excellence, communicate a strategic vision, and develop shared governance plans? How can you do the same? Identify and learn from people who have done a good job leading cross-functional and multilevel initiatives. Identify how your group can support other functions more effectively.

Mentoring Others

- Set up processes that make learning fluid and a part of the daily work.
- Talk with people to identify their learning styles, and tailor your mentoring activities to their styles.

Example:

Recognize how other departments might see a proposed change simply as an additional load. Brainstorm how to convince those other departments with nothing to gain from the change to take on the extra load. You might, for example, appeal to the nurses' service orientation—their desire to care for the patient and meet his or her needs. Recognize the other parties' situation and the extra steps the proposed change will cause. If the other parties need training to carry out the proposed change, help them obtain it. Model the way with your own mentoring.

Sharing Governance

- Set big-picture goals with your team, and then encourage them to work with their immediate team to determine specific plans and strategies for meeting those goals.

- Recognize the value of working together to provide the very best care for all patients.

Example:

State the challenge broadly, so that your team and the teams below them can determine the processes moving forward. A challenge like *"Together we mean something"* gives teams leeway to define what they believe needs to be done to improve care. Encourage leaders to form committees to formulate plans for meeting the goal within their own departments. Praise the efforts of teams working together to design new procedures for "best care" practices. Develop strategies for working with the reluctant few.

Implementing Plans

- Translate strategic priorities into concrete implementation steps and actions.
- Work with your team to determine how to track and measure success.

Example:

Design a kickoff session to get the buzz going and create some fun. Early on in the process, create forums to share information and capture lessons. Schedule meetings so that staff nurses can attend. True change happens at the unit level, and unit staff needs to see the results of their shared decision making. Hold regular meetings where you review process and go over deadlines. Encourage staff to return with suggestions for meeting the targets. Continuously celebrate both small and big wins—and everything in between.

Collaborating with Physicians

- Break down barriers that prevent collaboration, and watch for excessive territoriality.

- When trust is shaken, make good faith efforts to rebuild it by your own role modeling.

Example:

Doctors may perceive NPs' proposals to take on more responsibility as "power grabs." Have the patience to develop positive relationships with physicians and the skill to make physicians believe that the idea you are proposing will work for them and their patients. As one nurse aptly put it, "You must be willing to develop the relationships necessary to soothe fears and establish trust." Recognize that nurses and physicians share commonalities around perceived lack of respect and the weight of a consuming work life caring for others.

Developing Good Relationships

- Develop and nurture relationships with physicians and senior leaders.
- Understand the needs of others, and recognize the power of favors.

Example:

Get to know the physicians and senior leaders with whom you work. Learn what makes them happy and what frustrates them. Pay attention to timing when you approach them with critical concerns. Jump at opportunities to take on greater responsibility; doing so may expose you to even better opportunities. Remind those you do a favor for that you will expect them to reciprocate should you need their help down the road.

CHAPTER EIGHT

The Certified Registered Nurse Anesthetist: Reassuring Patients, Encouraging Cooperation in the Operating Room, and Documenting Patient Care

History of the Nurse Anesthetist

Nurse anesthetists have been providing anesthesia care in the United States for nearly 150 years. One of the first American nurses to provide anesthesia was Catherine Lawrence, who administered it during the American Civil War. The first "official" nurse anesthetist was Sister Mary Bernard, a Catholic nun who practiced in 1887 at St. Vincent's Hospital in Erie, Pennsylvania.[1]

The most famous nurse anesthetist was Alice Magaw, who worked at St. Mary's Hospital (later the Mayo Clinic) from 1899 to 1908. Dr. Charles Mayo gave Ms. Magaw the title "mother of anesthesia" for her many achievements, including mastery of the open-drop inhalation technique of anesthesia using ether and chloroform.[2] During Ms. Magaw's tenure at St. Mary's, Dr. Mayo and she published five articles on anesthesia and they both presented two of their papers before medical societies. Hundreds of physicians and nurses came to Minnesota from other states and around the world to learn from the pair about anesthesia practices.

After graduating from Boston City Hospital Training School for Nurses in 1900, Agatha Hodgins went to work at Lakeside Hospital in Cleveland, Ohio, and in 1908 began to work as an anesthetist for surgeon George Crile. Soon she was instructing other nurses in the administration of anesthesia. In 1914, she and Dr. Crile went to France with the American Ambulance Group to care for sick and wounded members of the Allied Forces.[3] While there, Hodgins taught physicians and nurses from England and France about administering nitrous oxide–oxygen anesthesia. On her return, she established the Lakeside Hospital School of Anesthesia. Graduates of her school dispersed throughout the United States. In 1931, Hodgins and many of her alumnae founded the National Association of Nurse Anesthetists, renamed the American Association of Nurse Anesthetists (AANA) in 1939.

About the AANA

Today the AANA represents more than 44,000 certified registered nurse anesthetists (CRNAs) and student registered nurse anesthetists nationwide. As advanced practice nurses, CRNAs administer more than 32 million anesthetics in the United States each year. The AANA developed and implemented a certification program in 1945, a mechanism for accreditation in 1952, and a recertification program in 1978. AANA has been a leader among professional organizations, supporting practice standards and guidelines and providing consultation to both private and governmental organizations.[4] Because of the AANA, research grants are available to students, faculty, and practicing CRNAs, and more than 90 percent of nurse anesthetists are members of the association. The CRNA credential is an indicator of both quality and competence.

- **AANA Vision Statement:** *AANA will be a preeminent professional association for healthcare and patient safety.*

- **AANA Mission Statement:** *AANA advances patient safety, practice excellence, and its members' profession.*

- **AANA Core Values:**
  - *Patient safety*
  - *Care for the whole patient, from a nursing perspective*
  - *Professional excellence and personal well-being*
  - *Healthcare policy and collaboration*

○ *Integrity and quality in all professional and clinical settings*

CRNAs in the Military

As noted earlier, nurses first provided anesthesia care to soldiers on the battlefields of the Civil War. Since World War I, nurse anesthetists have provided wounded troops with anesthetics in every war in which the United States has been engaged. CRNAs have provided 80 percent of all anesthetics given to U.S. military personnel in all branches of the service, including the Navy, Army, Marine Corps, and Air Force. These advanced practice nurses have suffered combat wounds, been held as prisoners of war, and lost their lives serving their country. The United States and foreign governments have honored them for outstanding achievements, dedication to duty, and treating the seriously wounded.[5] CRNAs provide care for all troops around the world, on ships, on the battlefield, in hospitals, in tents, and in Veteran's Administration hospitals.

CRNAs: Main Providers of Anesthesia Services in Rural Areas

CRNAs are the predominant providers of anesthesia services to the approximately 25 percent of the U.S. population that lives in rural areas. CRNAs perform 70 percent of the anesthesia care in rural hospitals, and 37 percent of CRNAs practice in towns with fewer than 50,000 residents.[6] Despite efforts to attract anesthesiologists to rural hospitals, there is little evidence of their commitment to practice in these hospitals. Community hospitals also have difficulty attracting CRNAs. Looking to the future, more than one quarter of todays CRNAs are expected to retire during the next 10–15 years. The vital role CRNAs play in these small rural hospitals must be recognized.[7]

CRNAs are the sole source of anesthesia care in many rural hospitals, where they administer anesthesia for less complicated surgical procedures. The communities these CRNAs serve seem satisfied with the services the CRNAs are providing, which speaks to the capability of CRNAs to function without anesthesiologist oversight.[8] In such areas as Charlevoix, Cheboygan, Harrisville, and Port Sanilac, Michigan, CRNAs are the only game in town. For example, at the Cheboygan Hospital, patients may receive all their anesthesia care from a CRNA yet assume they were being attended to by a physician.

> Mike Dosch, CRNA: *When I approach a patient in scrubs and a mask, the patient may assume that I am a doctor. This is especially true of older patients, and I have to correct them. However, in most cases I can deliver services that are not distinguishable for the patient.*

One CRNA's Story

Rosalyn Harrison, CRNA, DNAP grew up in the city of Detroit and received her associate's degree from Mercy College in 1989. After the merger of Mercy College and the University of Detroit, she went back to school and received her BSN and then on to anesthesia school to obtain her nurse anesthesia degree in 1995. Much later, she decided to go back to school and get her doctoral degree, finally graduating in 2012 with her Doctor of Nurse Anesthesia Practice (DNAP) degree.

> Rosalyn Harrison: *Currently, I'm employed full-time as a staff anesthetist at St. John Macomb—Oakland Hospital in Warren; I also have a contingent position at St. Mary's Hospital in Livonia and Troy Beaumont Hospital, in Troy, Michigan. Prior to that I was at St. John Riverview Hospital (SJDRH), which unfortunately closed in June 2007. While employed at SJDRH, I held the following positions: staff anesthetist, chief anesthetist, and interim director of Perioperative Services. I was responsible for overseeing the functions of the operating room to ensure that surgical services provided*

were efficient and met JACHO requirements to maintain a safe environment for our patients. Other responsibilities were to maintain adequate staffing and services outside of the OR, such as labor and delivery, interventional radiology and endoscopy. Patients and surgeons were our customers. My primary goal was to assure the needs of our customers were attended to and providing a safe and comfortable environment in our healthcare facility.

Easing Patient Fears of Anesthesia

Roz's first action is to review the patient's health history to make sure that she knows about the patient. She can then judge whether the proposed anesthetic is appropriate for the patient. Together, the CRNA and the anesthesiologist make the decision about the type of anesthetic to be administered. The surgeon is consulted on occasion as to what type of anesthesia is needed to perform the surgical procedure. Every detail counts, including the patient's cardiovascular, diabetes, and respiratory disease status. About twenty years ago, propofol (Diprivan) was introduced to anesthesia providers and sense then has replaced sodium thiopental (Pentothal). Patients are given probofol (deep sedation) or another drug such as midazolam/fentanyl (conscious sedation) for surgery.[9] Anesthesia providers find propofol to be beneficial; it wears off quickly and leaves no grogginess or nausea. (Patients who are prone to nausea can be given drugs to prevent its occurrence.) The goal in selecting an anesthetic is for patients to be comfortable, especially after the surgery. They should wake up with minimal grogginess.

CRNAs serve both critically ill and non-critical patients. Most patients are scheduled for elective surgery; while others are being treated for emergent situations.

Rosalyn Harrison: *What I practice, and what I hope that all nurse anesthetists practice, is treating patients the way they would like to be treated. If I were a patient, I would like only the best care delivered in a safe manner.*

Anesthesia providers typically do not interact with patients for an extended period of time; therefore, patients typically do not get a chance to know their providers. CRNAs assess patients, and then wheel them away to the operating room. The situation is different for a floor or a critical care nurse. Those nurses have a greater opportunity to establish a rapport/trusting relationship with their patients.

Rosalyn Harrison: *During the short time that I interact with the patient, I'm personable, show concern for the patient and try my best to alleviate any fears that the patient have prior to the surgery. Many patients are afraid of not waking up, especially after the incident with legendary Michael Jackson. Many patients inquire about propofol as to how the drug will impact them. I assure them that a fully trained and licensed anesthetist is administering the anesthesia and knows how to monitor patients while they receive anesthesia.*

I am a very pleasant person and keep a smile on my face 90 percent of the time. A smile goes a long way at a time when patients are fearful of the unknown and stressed about their upcoming surgery. I always try and make my patients feel at ease by introducing myself as their nurse anesthetist and informing them that, 'I will put them to sleep for surgery.' I will touch their arm softly if they feel it will help decrease their anxiety level. "Hello, my name is Roz, and I will be administering your anesthesia today during your surgery and monitoring you closely to make sure everything goes smoothly." I address the patient with a smile and ask whether he or she has any questions regarding anesthesia. "Is there anything I can do for you before we go to the operating room?" I then give the patient a warm blanket, which he or she seem to greatly appreciate once we enter the OR suite because the rooms are usually freezing.

If I see the patient's family, it is probably only five minutes before transporting the patient to the operating room. Some patients have very supportive families who want to ask about the anesthesia. I try my best to answer all of their questions and to help the family members feel at ease, rather than worried about their loved ones and what will happen as a result of the anesthesia.

Fostering Collaboration in the Operating Room

Individuals with diverse personalities will need to interact with each other in a cooperative manner in the operating room.[10] The members of Roz's team include surgeons, anesthesiologists, nurses, and surgical technicians. Most of the surgical team members have a good working relationship and have minimal conflict.

Rosalyn Harrison: *The anesthesiologist and the CRNA talk about the plan of care for our patient. If there is an area of concern, I feel comfortable about speaking up and discussing my concerns with the anesthesiologist because I am the patient's advocate. The safety of the patient is the number one priority. We discuss the anesthetic plan of care and determine which anesthetic is best for the patient depending on the patient's health status. In the end, we all come to an agreement regarding the safest anesthetic to provide for our patient.*

If the anesthesiologist is in the operating room, some surgeons treat the anesthetist as if she or he doesn't exist. The surgeon listens to the anesthesiologist and sometimes acts or pretends that the anesthetist is not in the room; however, if the anesthesiologist is not in the room, then the surgeon treats us with respect 90 percent of the time. Keep in mind that the anesthesiologist is often in the OR for only a brief period of time; however, if problems occur, we do not hesitate to call on our anesthesiologist, who will come into the room and provide council to help solve the problem. When cases go smoothly, we may not see the anesthesiologist at all.

Sometimes, when we have a critical case, everyone is on edge. You might hear a couple of voices being raised, but it is really nothing personal. We need to get the job done and do the very best for the patient safety. In the end, we all work together and collaborate as a team to provide a safe anesthetic for the patient.

Documenting Patient Care

Effectively documenting patient care includes legible penmanship and not leaving any check boxes blank.[11] The care that is provided is measured by patient outcomes, and also by the records kept at the end of the shift, the end of the week, and the end of the year. If it is not documented, that means it was not done.

Rosalyn Harrison: *If I do not check the box that verifies that both of the patient's arms were padded and the patient comes out of the OR with some sort of nerve injury, then I am at fault because an unchecked box means that a particular task was missed. The judge and the jury determine the verdict of a malpractice case dependent upon what is charted by the caregivers.*

The key thing about documentation is that all patient care must be measurable and thorough, including all medications. It is important that CRNAs learn to identify and produce good documentation, which is clear and concise and includes observations, nurses' actions and patient responses, and safety precautions taken to protect the patient.[12] Electronic medical records will be standard operating procedure in the future; when that time comes, all physicians, nurses, and staff members will need to use approved abbreviations.

Put down the date and time of the entry and sign it. Always make sure that each staff member verifies the information with the patient. The federal government wants every department to convert to electronic medical records. All hospitals will be required to go green by 2020.

Working Together to Create a Better Health Care Future

Michael Dosch, CRNA, PhD recounts the circuitous path he took to becoming a nurse anesthetist.

> Mike Dosch: *My father had been a general practitioner in Grayling, Michigan. I saw how hard he worked, with exhausting hours, too many patients, and no partners to pick up the slack. For a long time, none of us took more than two days of vacation at a time. I did not want to become a physician.*

After graduating from the University of Michigan in 1975, Mike went to work as a payments clerk for the welfare department, a job he did not find challenging and one that did not make him happy. However, he lived next door to two nurses, who liked their jobs, felt that they were doing important work, and believed that their profession gave them a lot of mobility. Mike volunteered at Mott Children's Hospital in Ann Arbor for six months and found that sick patients did not bother him. So he enrolled in nursing school in 1981 and received a diploma in nursing from Detroit's Mercy School of Nursing. After that, he worked for five years at Henry Ford Hospital as a floor nurse and then in the ICU.

Becoming a Male Nurse Anesthetist

Mike Dosch: [While I was working in the ICU], *I was introduced to the anesthesia program. I had not realized that male nurses even did that kind of work. So I took a couple of*

*years off and went back to school to get a master's of science
in nurse anesthesia, graduating in 1987, when I was almost
thirty-four years old. I have been working in anesthesia for
more than twenty years.*

Mike finds his work a lot of fun, very rewarding, very high
stress, and extremely important. He worked in a neurosurgery unit
at Henry Ford Hospital in Detroit; a neurosurgeon specializes in
operating on the brain, head, neck, and spinal cord. Originally, he
assumed that as a CRNA he would be around a lot of people who
were unconscious and that he would be really lonely. However, he
discovered that the job involves a lot of human contact.

Mike Dosch: *Patients in the operating room do not choose
their physicians, their nurse, or even sometimes, their surgeon.
They have no reason to trust you or feel confidence in you.
They have no history with you or any sort of relationship,
but they need your services. So you have to quickly develop a
rapport with them and let them know that you are confident,
competent, and intend to do the very best for them. The
only way they will trust you is if you show them that you
care about their feelings. Patients do not care if you have
been a good guy for the past ten years; they care about your
performance right now. You are only as good as your last
review. If you do a terrible job, that is all they will care
about.*

*Everyone works as part of a team, even if the patient
is asleep. In most operating rooms, nurses will hand the
surgeons their surgical instruments. The CRNA stands
behind the anesthesia unit; however, there is a surprising
amount of contact between nurses and surgeons. Sometimes,
the surgeon is delayed, and you need to be the entertainment
and distraction. This prevents the patient from thinking
about what he or she is about to undergo. It is a human
activity, probably more human than I ever expected.*

Dealing with Operating Room Pressures

The culture in the operating room is very, very cold, both physically and emotionally. The schedule trumps everything else, and there is a lot of production pressure to do as many surgeries as possible. Physicians are generally scheduled for surgeries in the morning and then office hours in the afternoon. Families waiting for loved ones in the surgical waiting room can feel the tension and pressure; the room has some of the worst seats in the hospital. Anything that can be done to shorten the families' stay in the waiting and recovery rooms is a good thing. Anything that slows things down is not so good.

> Mike Dosch: *We must never forget that we are dealing with human beings with human problems. I once watched a surgeon walk up to a stretcher with a person on it and say, "Is 'it' ready?" Not "Is the patient ready?" but "Is 'it'— the case—ready?" You cannot cry over every case in the operating room, because you might be less effective. You have to distance yourself, but some surgeons do not know when to turn the distancing off.*
>
> *The OR culture may not be a good safety culture because it is such a hurry-up culture. If someone is fumbling with something even a little bit, the surgeon might say, "Can we get this going, while we are still young?" Such thinking does not lead to a safety culture. Safety is going slow and repeating things a thousand times.*

Improving the Safety Culture of the OR

The world's worst airline accident can offer lessons for OR teams. The investigation of the 1977 Tenerife runway crash revealed that the primary cause of the accident was the captain of the KLM flight's taking off without clearance from Air Traffic Control (ATC). The investigation specified that the captain, Jacob Veldhuyzen van Zanten, did not intentionally take off without clearance; rather, he fully believed, due to misunderstandings between his flight crew and ATC, that he had been cleared for takeoff. The first officer, Klaas Meurs, may have been too intimidated to challenge the captain's conclusion, perhaps by saying something like this: *"Hey, Jacob, are you sure that we are supposed to be on this runway? I do not think that we are cleared."* The Dutch investigators placed a greater emphasis on this possibility than did their American and Spanish counterparts, [13] but ultimately KLM admitted that its crew was responsible for the accident, and the airline financially compensated the victims.

The OR culture can be equally intimidating. People can be afraid to speak up if they see something wrong.[14] Now, however, in addition to being very careful to verify the patient's identity, many surgical teams like Mike's do a timeout before every surgery. Everybody in the room speaks and introduces him or herself; it is hard to work with people if you do not know their names. Other team members will call you out if you are looking down at a piece of paper or doing anything that interferes with the discussion.

Working at Oakwood Hospital

Since 2005, Mike has worked as a CRNA at Oakwood Hospital and Medical Center in Dearborn, Michigan. He values the importance of these pre-surgery timeouts to the safety culture of the OR. Because lightning does strike every once in a while, and the results can be devastating, everyone stops what they are doing, gets their eyes on each other, and follows the script on the wall. Team members make sure they have the right equipment, talk about fire risk, and antibiotics. It is important to get everyone to talk to each other and take a breath. The goal is to make sure that everyone is ready to start before laying cold steel on the patient.

Mike Dosch: *I know a nurse who brought a female patient all the way into the operating room and the team was just about to anesthetize her when the surgeon rushed in to tell them that there were two Mary Smiths on the board that day—and this was the wrong Mary Smith. She was on the wrong table in the wrong operating room. That is why we continually ask patients who they are and what they are here for. We are not numskulls and are not confused. We just want to hear it from the patient.*

Years and years ago, before my wife gave much thought to wrong-site surgery, she came back from a break just as the surgical team was laying the patient on her side and painting her skin with iodine. The team was close to starting the operation. My wife feared she was going crazy, and started digging in the charts, trying to find the consent form, looking at the OR schedule, and looking at the X-rays. Although she was very timid, she knew she had to speak up. "Guys, something is wrong. The X-rays say it is the right kidney, but you have the left side up." The operating surgeon has never forgotten what a huge jam [my wife] got them out of. Things like this can happen because the surgeon may not enter the operating room until the patient is ready and the patient may not be recognizable with a tube down her throat, draped and on the table, and with her hair in a bonnet. Also, surgeons may only see their patient once before surgery and then not until after the surgery when the patient is back in a hospital bed.

Nursing management activities are critical, though some staff do not want to hear for the fourth time the location of the fire extinguisher in the room. Management has the responsibility of making sure team members take things seriously and to make sure that everyone in the operating room feels that the patient is being cared for in the right way. It is only too tempting, when under a great deal of pressure to get as much done as possible, to take some shortcuts. We all do this; however, there are certain red lines that we do not cross because it is not safe. With the relentless pressure to keep things moving, we sometimes come as close as possible to those lines without doing anything unsafe. Everyone needs to be reminded that what we do is dangerous and how important it is to take a timeout before each case to breathe.

Building a Team Culture

In the OR there might be five or six people standing hip to hip around the patient. When nurses and surgeons work this closely with one another over the years, it engenders a trusting relationship, one of collaboration and a deep faith in what teammates are doing. The bonds of trust are deep and long-lasting. The surgeons, who are in charge, would prefer to work with the same people every day and would prefer that their teammates never take a vacation, except when they do. Surgeons do not like to work with new people because they have to spend time telling them their preferences and what to do.

> Mike Dosch: *I have been working with general and orthopedic surgeons at Oakwood Hospital and Medical Center weekly, with maybe twenty surgeries a year, for each surgeon, over an eight-year span of time. When I am working with someone new, I have to think about what to say, what I want, and what he or she needs to do.*
>
> *Surgeons often host Christmas parties, where teammates and their spouses go out to a nice club for a meal and a few drinks. People can let their hair down and develop some close bonds, listen to a band, dance, and have a good time.*

In the operating room, part of the nurse anesthesia culture is to foster bonds without let these relationships get out of hand. Management has a role in keeping the culture above board and the bonds close. Interactions between team members can depend on their positions within the team. Mike might make a joke to one teammate that he would not say to a physician with whom he has a more formal relationship.

Mike Dosch: *There are many tough times in the OR when the patient is in serious trouble and perhaps on the verge of death. The surgeon is under stress to produce a positive result and cannot fall apart. That is not good for anyone. What is needed is for the team to work together cooperatively—nurses with physicians and CRNAs with the anesthesiologists. In life-or-death situations, the patient will get the best outcome possible when people work together cooperatively.*

We think of surgeons as calling the shots, which legally they do, but it is not that simple. The physician decides the overall plan, while the CRNA controls the patient's heartbeat, blood gases, and other vital signs during surgery and determines if the patient is getting too much or too little anesthesia.

Mike Dosch: *If the physicians know me, and I am uncomfortable with what the patient is going through, I may stop them and say, "Let's not do this. Let's do this other thing instead." I can get my way because they know me and trust what I have to say. You do not want to stop surgery every time you have a concern because that would not look good. CRNAs work closely with surgeons and that fosters a unique and close relationship. The anesthesiologist manages up to four operating rooms, with a CRNA in each, and he or she determines the care received or responds to potentially traumatic cases.*

How Increased Use of CRNAs Can Save $1.2 Billion

Currently there are approximately 40,000 anesthesiologists and 44,000 CRNAs practicing in the United States.[15] Both types of providers are critical to supplying patients with safe anesthesia services. Research and analysis indicate that CRNAs are less costly to train than anesthesiologists and can provide the same level of anesthesia care as anesthesiologists. The two professionals are interchangeable, with both capable of providing anesthesia for complicated services such as open-heart surgeries, and organ transplants. As the demand for healthcare increases, it makes sense to expand the number of CRNAs and permit them to practice to the full extent of their training—to contain costs while maintaining good-quality care.[16]

CRNAs work in three sites: hospitals (both inpatient and outpatient surgery), freestanding ambulatory surgery centers, and physician and dentist offices. In about 29 percent of all cases requiring anesthesia, anesthesiologists practice alone. In the remaining 71 percent of cases, CRNAs work as a team with an anesthesiologist, alone under a surgeon's supervision, or as a single individual in many rural hospitals. The Centers for Medicare and Medicaid Services (CMS) should return to the original intention of allowing nurse anesthetists to work independently of a surgeon's or an anesthesiologist's supervision, to improve the cost-effectiveness of care.[17] This will lead not only to more cost-effective care but will also free anesthesiologists from legal responsibilities for patient care. In fact, surgeons and some anesthesiologists fully support CRNAs, and both professions contribute to the other and both raise each other up.[18]

Certified teachers are hard to come by because of the shortage of nurse educators and the growing number of students seeking admission to nursing schools. The primary barrier to increasing the number of training programs is lack of clinical access, and one of the barriers is a bias in the Medicare system that favors physician supervision of anesthesiology residents over nurse anesthetist students. Another potential barrier is a shortage of CRNA educators in universities and hospitals. Increasing the role of CRNAs in the administration of anesthesia would result in a significant savings to society, cutting costs by 16 percent of the nation's total anesthesia bill.[19] Congress cannot afford to stand by while nurse anesthesia programs are closed and replaced by anesthesiology residency programs.

CRNA Salaries

For CRNAs, the money is great, and prospects for job growth are excellent. In 2011 the average salary of male CRNAs was $171,700, down from an average of $175,000 in 2010, whereas the average salary for female CRNAs was $160,680, up from an average of $156,100 in 2010. Overall the 2011 average annual CRNA salary was $168,998.[20] Hospitals can save money by employing CRNAs: the average salary for anesthesiologists is $337,163.[21] The demand for CRNAs will increase as hospitals and group practices seek to save money while maintaining excellent patient care in the operating room and at group practices. However, CRNAs' responsibilities can be extremely stressful, especially in rural hospitals where they must be on call and ready to go at a moment's notice.

> Profile of a CRNA
> - 49% male
> - 51% female
> - 26% employed in a group practice
> - 60% employed by a hospital

The Educational Pathway to a CRNA

In the United States, aspiring CRNAs must first complete a bachelor's degree in a science-related field or a bachelor of science in nursing (BSN). Then, they must be licensed by passing the NCLEX-RN, the national licensing exam. Once licensed, most RNs are required to have one to two years of full-time experience in an acute care setting, such as a surgical intensive care unit or medical intensive care. Following the acute care experience, nurses apply to the graduate degree-granting program accredited by the Council on Accreditation (COA). The graduate degree in nurse anesthesia can run anywhere from 24 to 36 months. It takes the average person 7–13 years from start to finish to become a CRNA.

Education is offered at a master's degree or a doctoral program and requires prerequisites similar to those for medical school. All programs provide students with the scientific, clinical, and professional foundations upon which to establish safe clinical practices. Students study statistics and scientific inquiry and participate in student- and faculty-generated research. Clinical residencies afford supervised experiences for students to learn anesthesia techniques, test their theories, and apply their knowledge to clinical issues. Students work with patients of all ages who require medical, surgical, obstetric, dental, and pediatric interventions.[22]

Nurse Anesthetist School Requirements at a Glance[23]

- Bachelor of science in nursing (BSN)
- Registered nursing license
- 1–2 years critical care/ICU experience
- Cumulative GPA of 3.0 or better
- Combined minimum GRE score of 1,000 or better
- TOEFL (Test of English as a Foreign Language) as applicable
- Certifications (BLS, ACLS, PALS)
- Prerequisite classes
- Other standard requirements

Actions for CRNAs

Question for Reflection

How are you creating an atmosphere of calm and collaboration in the operating room? Teamwork is important, especially with the ICU nurses, the surgeon, residents, and physician assistants. What are you doing to center the team and get them ready for the operation?

Earning Loyalty and Trust

- What steps are you taking to earn the loyalty of your peers, including surgeons, residents, and ICU nurses?
- When you commit to something, you do it. That means a lot to those you work with because they put a lot of trust in you.

Example:

Surgeons and ICU nurses can often be stressed out during particularly difficult surgeries. Although the nurse anesthetist is focused on the job at hand, entering the room with a positive attitude can help everyone in the room settle down. Bring your own high standards to your work, and expect the same of others so that your patients receive the best of care.

Going Over Protocols[24]

- Work like a nurse, but think like a reporter. Think about what needs to be documented: key events, treatments, and procedures.
- Realize the value of documentation, and learn to identify good documentation.

Example:

Talk to patients and their families, and teach them what to expect during the operation. Go over each protocol until the patient and the family indicate that they understand. Good documentation includes observations, nurse's actions, patient's response, unusual incidents, omitted treatments, and safety precautions. Your documentation is an action plan for good care.

Research and the CRNA

- Be educated about the latest research, and incorporate the research results into good patient care.
- Work closely with surgeons and nurses to monitor the amount of anesthesia the patient receives and makes adjustments as necessary.

Example:

Understand how the latest research can impact patient care and incorporate the research into safety protocols. Emphasize research to expand the profession's knowledge base and to establish an evidence-based practice. CRNAs need to participate in and fulfill the AANA vision as recognized leaders in anesthesia research by removing barriers and strengthening the educational curricula.[25]

Collaborating as a Team in the Operating Room

- Apply your teaching skills to medical students, nurses, and residents by guiding them while allowing them to practice and learn.
- Understand the requirements of each role on the surgical team and how those responsibilities affect the patient's outcome.

Example:

Use a checklist to adhere to critical management steps during the operation. Checklists can improve operating room safety. Be honest about mistakes; people should not be punished for them. Stop when you feel that you have made an error, acknowledge it, and talk about it in a nonpunitive way. Be honest by putting the patient first and setting your own ego aside.

Creating Great Students

- Select classes that are meaningful, practical, and pertinent to what you plan to do after graduation.[26]
- Recognize that the faculty has lots of experience and takes teaching very seriously. Take advantage of small class sizes to request individual attention and of your faculty's high standards and focus on making you successful.

Example:

In one program, students work in 21 community locations and volunteer eight hours in community settings. Every year some students join a medical mission to provide treatment to patients in third-world countries. Infuse your work with a sense of mission, intellect, and drive. Have a sense of humility about what you do, so that every day, with every patient you encounter, you do not take anything for granted.

CHAPTER NINE

One Nurse's Story of Professional Transformation—Breast Cancer Treatment Specialist, Menopause Practitioners and Nursing Issues Writer

Dr. Lisa Chism received her bachelor of science in nursing (RN) and a master of science in nursing (GNP), and then received a post-master's fellowship (WHNP) from the University of Michigan. She went on to earn her doctor of nursing practice (DNP) from Rochester, Michigan's Oakland University in 2007. Earning a DNP was a personal goal for Lisa, who was one of the first NPs to apply to the DNP program.

Lisa began her practice at Wyandotte Hospital and Medical Center, where she worked from 1990 to 1994. In 1994 to 1995, she moved to General Medicine PC, a group of board-certified physicians and nurse practitioners specializing in geriatrics, physical medicine, and rehabilitation.[1] It was there that she learned about geriatric care, a focus that she maintains to this day. From 1996 to 2002 she was affiliated with American Geriatric Consultants. From 2002 to 2007, she worked at Livonia Family Physicians, PC and then moved on to Beaumont Hospital's department of internal medicine, where she worked from 2007 to 2009.[2]

Geriatric medicine requires plenty of patience and a real emphasis on taking care of the aging. Together with physicians, Lisa has what it takes to listen carefully, hold hands with a geriatric patient, and consider what is best for her or him. Geriatric care focuses on the patient and the patient's family by providing the information they need to make crucial decisions about quality of care rather than length of life. Lisa and physicians work closely with patients and families, helping them decide what type of care they wish to receive and which options are best for their particular condition. With joint preparation in both geriatrics and women's health, Lisa took the leap and entered Oakland University's doctor of nursing practice program in 2009.

> *What we have done for ourselves alone dies with us; what we have done for others and the world remains and is immortal.*
> —Albert Pike

Lisa chose the DNP as a personal goal because it provided the opportunity to focus on practice rather than research. As a result of her DNP, she has become well-versed in new ways to treat her patients. She attributes her engagement in nursing education, focus on clinical aspects of care, and achievements in policy and leadership to her experience working toward her DNP. When Lisa first spoke to other nurses about the DNP, some scoffed at the idea. When she promotes the DNP today, however, she finds most audiences far more receptive to the concept.

Lisa Chism: *The DNP brought me back to nursing as a discipline and practice. I became better versed in adopting different ways to look at patient and family care.*

Lisa joined the Barbara Ann Karmanos Cancer Institute (affiliated with Wayne State University's School of Medicine) in 2009, as a nurse practitioner in the Alexander J. Walt Comprehensive Breast Center Women's Wellness Clinic. She is a member of the Karmanos Center's Breast Multidisciplinary Team, a certified menopause practitioner, and a member of the Patient Education, Membership, and Scientific Programming committees for the North American Menopause Society (NAMS).[3] She is also an active preceptor and adjunct faculty at Madonna University in Livonia and the University of Michigan.

In 2011 Lisa was honored with induction as a fellow of the

American Academy of Nurse Practitioners (AANP), the only full-service professional membership organization in the United States for NPs of all specialties. As a fellow, Lisa's responsibilities are to promote the NP role, mentor future NP leaders, and contribute to the profession locally, nationally, and globally.

Lisa Chism: *Personally, I am honored and humbled by my . . . induction as a fellow of AANP. This recognition validates my contributions to the profession, as well as my long-term commitment to nursing and the role of the nurse practitioner.*

At the AANP Conference in June 2012, Lisa and Diane Todd Pace, PhD, APRN, BC, CCD, NCMP, FAANP presented a three-hour workshop on menopause. Dr. Pace is an assistant professor, Acute and Chronic Care Department, at the University of Tennessee's Health Science Center College of Nursing in Memphis. She was inducted in 2007 as an AANP fellow for outstanding efforts in clinical practice, patient advocacy, and professional/political leadership. Diane is a certified menopause practitioner (1991) through NAMS[4] and is a member of the American Nurses Association and the Tennessee Nurses Association. In their menopause workshop, Drs. Chism and Pace covered such topics as hormone therapy, atrophic vaginitis,[5] and the development of a menopause curriculum for the Association of Professors of Gynecology and Obstetrics (APGO). Dr. Chism was appointed as the NAMS's 2011 certified menopause practitioner, which she considers a great honor.[6]

Lisa has written *The Doctor of Nursing Practice: A Guidebook for Role Development and Professional Issues* (2009, updated 2013).[7] She also publishes a bimonthly column, titled "DNP Perspectives," in the *Advance for NPs and PAs* magazine. Lisa has also developed a nursing theory, called "Chism's Middle-Range Spiritual Empathy Theory," to explain the relationship between nurses' spiritual care perspective and their expressions of spiritual empathy. Lisa set out to demonstrate how a middle-range theory was developed and tested through research that *"examined relationships between nurse-expressed empathy and two patient outcomes: patient-perceived empathy and patient distress."*[8]

Lisa Chism: *Little attention has been given to identifying the caring, empathic processes nurses might use to promote the spiritual well-being of their patients. Also, it is unclear to what extent the spiritual care perspectives of nurses affect their ability to express spiritual empathy. This theory-driven, descriptive correlational study examined the relationship between student nurses' spiritual care perspectives and their expressions of spiritual empathy. Findings of this study suggest that clinically, a self-reflective approach to evaluating one's own spiritual care perspectives should be undertaken before attempting to implement empathic, caring processes.*[9]

Lisa divided study nurses into three groups and studied nurses' spiritual care perspective toward patients and how that perspective impacts nurses' ability to convey empathy. The study showed that DNP practitioners, most in their early fifties, expressed the most empathy of the three groups.

> It isn't until you come to a spiritual understanding of who you are—not necessarily a religious feeling, but deep down, the spirit within—that you can begin to take control.
>
> —Oprah Winfrey

Lately, Lisa has been involved in developing a practice through the Women's Wellness Clinic at an additional location—the Lawrence and Idell Weisberg Cancer Treatment Center in Farmington Hills, Michigan. Lisa notes that at both the Detroit and Farmington Hills locations:[10]

Karmanos offers specialists in breast cancer and highly trained nurse practitioners who are focused on overall breast health and wellness. The clinic offers guidance, support, and screenings for women with a history of breast cancer, those who have a genetic predisposition for breast cancer, or those who have general concerns or questions about their own breast health.

The goal of the Women's Wellness Clinic is to offer another level of care to women concerned about their breast health, while working closely with their current doctors to keep everyone informed about their care. Whether a woman wants to schedule a mammogram or have her risk for breast cancer evaluated, we are here to offer these and other services.

As an advocate for NPs, one of the areas that Lisa has focused on is advocating for different ways to bill for services. Lisa became involved in advocating for increased credentialing with additional carriers within her institution and alternative ways to bill for services rendered to breast cancer, menopausal and geriatric women.

People go through challenging moments of losing people and having their life threatened from illness and real grief. But they get through it. And that's testament to the human spirit, and its—we are fragile, but we are also divine.

—Sheryl Crowe.

Having completed the DNP program, Lisa feels increased dedication to her profession and a greater satisfaction about future career goals. As a result of her DNP, she was motivated to write a book, become certified in menopause (passing the same test that physicians take), develop the menopause clinic, and published articles on menopause and breast cancer. She now has her eye on taking a sexual health seminar through the University of Michigan Health System.[11] With this additional knowledge, Lisa plans to investigate the relationship between having breast cancer, experiencing menopause, and expressing one's sexual awareness.

She has become a cheerleader for the profession of nursing, focused her goals, increased her feelings of empowerment, and developed trust in her relationships with physicians, fellow nurses, students, and her staff. Her consultative experience includes being on the DNP Advisory Board for the University of Detroit–Mercy and the Norvo Nordisk Advisory Board on Atrophic Vaginitis Treatments. She is a member of the NAMS's Consumer Education Committee 2010–2011 and 2011–2012, the NAMS Membership Committee 2012–2013, and the NAMS's Scientific Planning Committee 2011–2012 and 2012–2013.

Moving from an RN to a DNP Degree

The doctor of nursing practice (DNP) is a terminal professional degree that focuses on the clinical aspects of nursing rather than academic research. The curriculum for the DNP degree includes advanced nursing practice, health policy, leadership, research methodology, information technology, and population health.[12]

In 2004, the American Association of Colleges of Nursing (AACN) recommended that all nurses seeking credentials as a nurse practitioner seek a DNP degree with the phase-in date of 2015. Loretta Ford, NP, cofounder of the nurse practitioner role, describes the DNP as *"the next logical step towards clinical excellence, leadership and political acumen in advanced practice nursing. The environments in which practice occurs demand leaders with vision, knowledge, communication skills, political savvy and a sense of social justice beyond that required for the one-to-one relationship of patient care."*[13]

DNP programs must follow certain standards by 2015 for their graduates to be eligible for certification as NPs. These "essentials" include addressing emerging healthcare needs, leadership skills, social justice concerns, and a vision for the future of healthcare in America. Most DNP programs start with the master's of science in nursing (MSN) and refrain from addressing education requirements in the master's program. Generally the programs take approximately two years and around 40 credit hours, though programs may vary depending upon the school. Nurses graduating from a bachelor of science in nursing (BSN) program may also apply, but it is generally recommended that these nurses gain some experience in a hospital or clinic before moving on to the DNP. For a BSN nurse to attain the DNP degree requires two years full time or four years part time and 79–82 credit hours.

Why Move to the DNP?[14]

- *The changing demands of this nation's complex healthcare environment require the highest level of scientific knowledge and practice expertise to assure quality patient outcomes. The Institute of Medicine, Joint Commission, Robert Wood Johnson Foundation, and other authorities have called for reconceptualizing educational programs that prepare today's health professionals.*

- *Some of the many factors building momentum for change in nursing education at the graduate level include the rapid expansion of knowledge underlying practice; the increased complexity of patient care; national concerns about the quality of care and patient safety; shortages of nursing personnel, which demand a higher level of preparation for leaders who can design and assess care; shortages of nursing faculty with doctorate degrees; and increasing educational expectations for the preparation of other members of the healthcare team.*

- *In a 2005 report titled* Advancing the Nation's Health Needs: NIH Research Training Programs, *the National Academy of Sciences called for nursing to develop a non-research clinical doctorate to prepare expert practitioners who can also serve as clinical faculty. The American Association of Colleges of Nursing's work to advance the DNP is consistent with this call to action.*

- *Nursing is moving in the direction of other health professions in the transition to the DNP. Medicine (MD), dentistry*

(DDS), pharmacy (PharmD), psychology (PsyD), physical therapy (DPT), and audiology (AudD) all offer practice doctorates.

There are 184 DNP Programs currently enrolling students with 101 programs in the planning stages.

- *At schools of nursing across the United States, 184 DNP programs are currently enrolling students; an additional 101 DNP programs are in the planning stages.*

- *DNP programs now exist in 40 states plus the District of Columbia. States with more than five programs include Florida, Massachusetts, Minnesota, New York, Pennsylvania, and Texas.*

- *From 2010 to 2011, the number of students enrolled in DNP programs increased from 7,034 to 9,094. During that same period, the number of DNP graduates increased from 1,282 to 1,595.*

- *For a comprehensive list of DNP programs, please see the list in the Appendix.*

DNP Essentials: Requirements for DNP Programs

1. **Scientific underpinnings for practice:** Programs must provide adequate content on life processes and functions of the body.

2. **Organizational and systems leadership for quality improvement and systems thinking:** DNP graduates must be knowledgeable about patients on individual population and community levels to help create new health care delivery models.

3. **Clinical scholarship and analytical methods for evidence-based practice:** DNP graduates must be able to put research into practice.

4. **Information systems/technology and patient care technology for the improvement and transformation of health care:** DNP graduates should know how to evaluate programs and information systems to best care for patients and to evaluate ethical and legal issues surrounding health care technology.

5. **Health care policy for advocacy in health care:** DNP programs should prepare graduates to take on leadership roles in political actions to promote patient care as well as the nursing profession.

6. **Interprofessional collaboration for improving patient and population health outcomes:** DNP programs should contain content that prepares students for working on and creating collaborative health teams.

7. **Clinical prevention and population health for improving the nation's health:** DNP graduates should be able to provide risk reduction and illness prevention for patients and families as well as the entire population.

8. **Advanced nursing practice:** DNP programs should provide education for mastery in one specialty area of nursing practice.

Source: American Association of Colleges of Nursing. The Essentials of Doctoral Education for Advanced Practice Nursing. Issued October 2006. Available at http://www.aacn.nche.edu/DNP/pdf/Essentials.pdf

Admission Requirements for One Doctor of Nursing Practice (DNP) Program

The ideal candidate for Duke University School of Nursing's doctor of nursing practice program has excellent collegiate GPAs, is making an impact on nursing practice, and has leadership skills.[15]

Admission Criteria for Applicants with a BSN
- Earned BSN from a nationally accredited program
- GPA 3.0 or above on a 4.0 scale
- The GRE is waived if an applicant's cumulative undergraduate GPA is 3.4 or higher. Satisfactory performance on the GRE is required if your cumulative GPA is below 3.4
- Resume or CV
- Current licensure as a registered nurse in the state in which practice will occur
- Undergraduate statistics course
- Transcripts from all post-secondary institutions
- Three letters of reference pertaining to academic ability, professional competency, and personal character
- Personal statement
- E-portfolio of professional practice that highlights educational, professional, and community activities, as well as scholarship
- Telephone or in-person interview may be a part of the admission process

Admission Criteria for Applicants with an MSN (earned master's in nursing in an advanced nursing practice specialty from a nationally accredited program)
- Certification as an advanced practice nurse (if applicable)
- GPA 3.0 or above on a 4.0 scale
- Resume or CV
- Current licensure as a registered nurse in the state in which practice will occur
- Graduate inferential statistics course

- Graduate research methodology course
- Transcripts from all post-secondary institutions
- Three letters of reference pertaining to academic ability, professional competency, and personal character
- Personal statement
- E-portfolio of professional practice that highlights educational, professional, and community activities, as well as scholarship
- Telephone or in-person interview may be a part of the admission process

DNP Class Time Requirements for University of Michigan–Flint Program

BSN – DNP Program[16]

- Intended for bachelor's-prepared RNs who wish to pursue a DNP
- 2-year, full-time course or 4-year, part-time program
- Requires 79–82 credit hours
- Clinical courses are arranged in your area, making it convenient for you to gain practical experience

MSN – DNP Program

- Intended for master's- prepared nurses who are already certified nurse practitioners, nurse midwives, clinical nurse specialists, or certified registered nurse anesthetists
- 2-year, full-time course or 4-year, part-time course
- Requires 31–33 credit hours
- Clinical courses are arranged in your area, making it convenient for you to gain practical experience

Online DNP[17] Programs

- Programs conducted primarily online allow busy nursing professionals to work and study simultaneously.

- Most require periodic campus visits for symposia, 1,000 clinical hours, and a 1-year residency.
- Full-time study allows for completion of the DNP in 2 years; there is also a 4-year, part-time course.

Nursing Schools and Faculty Shortages

In Benner's stages of clinical competence a nurse passes through five levels of proficiency: novice, advanced beginner, competent, proficient, and expert.[18] However, the education of nurses is lagging the demand, and nursing schools are turning away tens of thousands of good applicants because of budget constraints and faculty shortages. Patients need good care from competent nurses with a focus on both clinical and empathetic care. Nurses at the various stages of Benner's clinical competence continuum must be enabled to move from taking orders to achieving a rare balance of nurses taking care of patients and patients seeing themselves in the eyes of the nurse.

Within the next ten years, half of nursing school faculty members will reach retirement age.[19] Even though the number of graduates from DNP programs remains fixed at about 8,000 per year, the demand for faculty stays high. To qualify for a faculty or APRN position, many nurses have to return to school and obtain additional academic degrees. Medicare is the largest single source of federal support for nursing education, yet the majority of funding goes to pre-professional education in nursing. Graduate education, including the preparation of NPs, does not qualify for reimbursement.[20] Incomes for nurses in the clinical setting and administration are higher than those of most nursing faculty, making it even more difficult to recruit faculty.[21]

Yet the demand for APNs continues to grow and may escalate further in light of the projected shortage of physicians and the 80-hour residency rule. The number of graduations from accredited NP programs peaked in 1998 at 8,199, falling since that time to

6,900. Faculty shortages and lack of financial assistance may deter many aspiring NPs from pursuing their DNP degree.

Nursing education needs a unified strategy for creating a nursing workforce sufficient in both numbers and education to meet the nation's healthcare needs. In an economy where jobs are scarce, it makes no sense to allow good nursing jobs to go unfilled because students are being turned away from nursing schools. New public funding is needed to help nursing schools expand educational opportunities for new nurses and those in other professions who want to go back to school for retraining. For example, during a conference on healthcare jobs, two women spoke of their experiences transitioning from a banking career and a career at Chrysler to the healthcare field. Transitions take time, but those who trust in themselves and are willing to work hard will find the right path.

CHAPTER TEN

Moving Healthcare Forward: The Role of the Advanced Practice Nurse (APN)

As APNs grow and learn more about the complexities of patient care, they develop practice skills and insights from experience.[1] With experience comes a heightened grasp of patient feelings and a deeper understanding of illnesses, which in turn guide the APN's actions. The APN's responses to patients become more caring as she or he moves from rule-bound thinking to a more intuitive grasp of the situation. Good APNs hone their skills as they develop a rich sense of the possibilities of good practice and excellent patient care. The expert nurse integrates theory and practice in multiple ways to create new possibilities for proficient care.

The "calling" that brings most nurses into the profession involves caring for patients, valuing other nurses, and sharing information. What detracts from that calling includes a high-paced, technology-driven environment, heavy patient loads, task-oriented medical practices, and pure exhaustion.[2] Practitioners and health system administrators grasp that a radical change is needed to reverse the reduction in caring that many nurses witness every day in hospitals and other healthcare delivery systems. Today nurses and health practitioners strive to establish caring relationships in which love, kindness, and sensitivity transform their interactions with patients and the public. Nurses participate in a process through which they connect with their patients human to human as well as spiritually. They combine the touch of a hand and genuine patient interaction with the critical medical-clinical aspects of their work.

Increasingly, caring practitioners depend upon relationships, partnerships, negotiations, communication patterns, and truly authentic connections. They are shifting toward spiritual care and the development of creative solutions to transcend the conventional medical/clinical/fix-it model of care. Nurses need to find their own source of inner peace and tranquility; they need to reexamine the medical model and search for their own values. Cost efficiency, quality clinical care, and patient caring can coexist. They are not mutually exclusive.

One Answer: The Medical Home Model

The American Academy of Pediatrics (AAP) introduced the medical home in 1967 as a way to take care of children with special needs. Since that time, the concept has grown tremendously into the medical home model. Principles surrounding the medical home model include a personal physician for each individual; a physician-directed medical practice; a process designed to take care of the whole patient with coordinated care, quality, and safety; enhanced prevention; and adequate provider payments.[3] The ideal medical home health system consists of multiple providers, each communicating with and accountable to each other, to coordinate and deliver high-quality care. In the medical home model participating physicians are paid a per-member-per-month care management fee in addition to regular fee-for-service payments.

How the Medical Home Model
Can Change Healthcare

There are four reasons why the medical home model makes sense as the United States moves forward with healthcare reform.[4]

1. **Cost Control.** The patient centered medical home (PCMH) model places cost containment at the center of its mission. The cost of healthcare continues to skyrocket; however, there is growing evidence that the PCMH model improves access to healthcare provider teams while at the same time

controlling costs.[5] The PCMH model provides incentives for efficiency but not at the expense of quality care.

The evidence also shows that primary care (in contrast to specialty care) is associated with a more equitable distribution of health in populations, a finding that holds in both cross-national and within-national studies. The means by which primary care improves health have been identified, thus suggesting ways to improve overall health and reduce differences in health across major population subgroups.[6]

2. **Cost Reductions Related to Care Standards.** Peter Orszag, during his tenure as director of the White House Office of Management and Budget, stated before the U.S. Senate Committee on Finance that our current approach to healthcare perpetuates a system in which 46 million uninsured people do not receive good care and puts an unnecessary burden on state governments.[7] Redirecting money to the medical home will both increase health and decrease health expenditures, reducing spending on unnecessary health services.

    The PCMH model is fast becoming a catalyst for health reform efforts across the country, and demonstration projects are appearing in almost every state. In the next few years, thousands of primary care practices will attempt to convert their offices into holistic, team-oriented practices with the focus directly on the patient. The PCMH model calls for innovative, relationship-centered patient care, reimbursement reform, use of new information technology, and heightened attention to chronic care.

3. **Coordination of Care.** Disease management programs often have disappointing results because they rarely integrate primary care physicians into the model. Patients often perceive these programs as designed purely for cost control, not care management. Often primary care physicians do not even know about the program until their patients tell

them they have been contacted. Then it is too late for the physician to endorse the program, and it discourages patient participation.

Transforming practices to a PCMH model requires a fundamental re-imagining, replacing old patterns of practice with new ones. The transformation will require new scheduling, new coordination with other parts of the healthcare system, quality improvement efforts, the development of team-based care, new ways for patient engagement, and fundamental changes in how practices are managed. The PCMH must be structured to enhance the patient experience. It requires fundamental transformation, not incremental change.[8]

4. **Patient/Physician Alignment.**

More physicians are switching from a for-profit service to nonprofit healthcare; they care more about living a balanced life than about both running a business and practicing medicine. This trend better aligns the patient, the physician, and nurse practitioners and improves preventive medicine. Redirecting money to the medical home model produces healthier people, reduces healthcare activities, and lowers spending on excessive services. Patient-centered care uses a team-based approach to provide a panoply of healthcare services for all life stages and situations, including acute care, chronic conditions, behavioral and mental health, prevention, and end-of-life care.

Healthcare Reimbursement and NPs

On the subject of reimbursement for healthcare services as it relates to NPs, the NP Roundtable recommends the following actions:[9]

- *Support efforts that increase patient access to the full primary care provider workforce, and allow for patient choice in provider selection.*

- *Re-engineer reimbursement systems to reflect the true costs of care to ensure that all practice settings, including primary care practices, nurse-managed health centers, and emerging delivery models, can be self-sustaining.*

- *Promote reimbursement based on services provided.*

- *Track provider-specific services and outcomes; linking outcomes to specific providers will promote accountability in care.*

- *Recognize outcomes of care as critical indicators in effective reimbursement models.*

- *Include nurse practitioner–led practices and nurse practitioners as full partners in medical homes, accountable care organizations (ACOs), insurance exchanges, and other developing innovations.*

- *Continue to remove the outdated legislative and regulatory barriers that impede the utilization of nurse practitioners to the top of their education and abilities in addressing patient care needs.*

One Nurse's Effort to Change Billing Practices

Deana Hays is a Family Nurse Practitioner, and Director of NP Programs and Adjunct Faculty, Oakland University School of Nursing. Deana set out to change the way billing was done at her workplace by working together with physicians to coordinate and integrate billing practices. Despite the rhetoric of NPs taking over for primary care physicians, the two work best when they work together. Physicians are a key piece of the program; without them

NPs cannot function effectively. Each member of the team of which Deana is a part (physicians, NPs, other health professionals) needed to identify how the practice impacted him or her professionally. Everyone was successful because they all shared one vision, functioned as a team, empowered each other, and worked together for both the patients and the organization.

Deana Hays: *The role of the nurse practitioner in primary care is becoming increasingly popular with the passage of the Patient Protection and Affordable Care Act. I recently attended a large conference with other NP faculty and providers where the American Association of Retired Persons (AARP) pointed out that the government does not recognize how much care NPs provide because they are billing under physician provider numbers rather than their own.*

Billing under a physician provider number meant the practice received 100 percent reimbursement for NP services provided rather than the 85 percent reimbursement it would have received if we had billed under our own numbers. What this essentially meant was that in the eyes of Medicare and private insurance companies it was the physician providing the care rather than the NPs. So I pushed the envelope because I found this [billing] practice to undermine the services that NPs work so hard to provide. This was not about money but about principle. The clinic was owned by a large healthcare system, so we [NPs] went to the legal and risk management department to determine if this practice was acceptable and found it was not.

Insurance companies (particularly Medicare) require NPs to bill under their own provider numbers. Through the proper channels and many, many meetings with the legal department, physicians, and managers, we were able to get the NPs to start billing under their own provider numbers. In my clinic we found that the NPs were providing more preventive services and seeing more patients than our physician colleagues. In order for the NPs to be successful in getting the health system and physicians to allow us to bill under our own provider numbers, we had to work together. We met collectively with the physicians, and since the physicians were employees of the organization, they were not affected by the NPs billing under their own provider numbers in the primary care clinics. In the end, NPs can now bill under their own provider numbers and get credit for the primary care services they are providing.

NPs Embrace the PCMH Model but Call for Care Model Diversity

Angela Golden, president of the American Academy of Nurse Practitioners (AANP), issued this statement concerning the American Academy of Family Physicians' (AAFP's) report, *Primary Care for the 21ˢᵗ Century: Ensuring a Quality, Physician-led Team for Every Patient:*[10]

The American Academy of Nurse Practitioners strongly supports patient-centered and team-based care models. However, AANP believes that AAFP's efforts to link these evolving models of care with the licensure of nurse practitioner (NP) practice are misdirected and out of step with today's environment. More specifically, AAFP's position is directly contrary to the recommendations of the Institute of Medicine and the National Council of State Boards of Nursing. In fact, the requirements for physician-leadership of a health care home, as proposed by the AAFP, is inconsistent with the requirements set by the National Committee for Quality Assurance (NCQA), URAC Accreditation, and the Joint Commission, each a well-known and respected organization currently accrediting patient-centered health care homes led by NPs.

As our nation looks to address health care provider

workforce challenges, we must embrace the diversity of care models that multiple disciplines sharing overlapping knowledge and skills can offer our country. For nearly half a century, NPs have been providing quality of care and offering increased health care access to millions of patients. More than 100 studies analyzing care provided by NPs and physicians have demonstrated that NPs have the same or better patient outcomes when compared to physicians. Making full use of the NP workforce is a critical piece of a multi-pronged solution to address the urgent need for health care access in our nation. The ongoing attempts by the AAFP to limit the ability of NPs to practice to the full extent of their education and training only serves to increase the already overwhelming hardships placed on millions of Americans who are struggling to gain access to high quality health care.

America needs to embrace a healthcare system that allows advanced practice providers to treat simple problems, primary care physicians to treat more complex problems, and specialists to treat only the most complex conditions. APNs in partnership with physicians and other providers need to move forward with evidence-based, collaborative models of delivery to promote

How One Nurse Helped Start a Dialysis Center

The U.S. Renal Data System estimates that the number of people in American experiencing kidney failure doubled from 2003 to 2010, growing from about 320,000 to 650,000 patients.[11] Healthy kidneys clean blood by removing excess fluid, minerals, and wastes. They also make hormones that keep bones strong and blood healthy. When kidneys fail, harmful wastes build up in the body, the blood pressure rises, and the body retains excess fluid and fails to make enough red blood cells. When this happens, treatment to replace the work of failed kidneys is necessary.

There are several ways of making up for failing kidneys. The filtering job can be replaced by a kidney transplant or dialysis. There are two types of dialysis, hemodialysis and peritoneal dialysis. Hemodialysis uses an "artificial kidney" machine to pump blood through a filter that mimics the function of a human kidney. Treatments are usually done at a dialysis clinic, 3 times a week for about 3 to 4 hours.

Peritoneal dialysis (PD) uses the patients' peritoneal membrane as a filter for the blood. A special fluid called dialysate is put into the patients' abdomen where it draws out water and waste through the peritoneal membrane. The dialysate is later drained out and replaced with fresh fluid. Treatments, also called "exchanges", are done daily or nightly at home. PD gives the patient more control because a scheduled dialysis session at a center is unnecessary. The PD patient can do treatments at home, at work, or on trips.

This independence makes it especially important for the patient to work closely with the health care team: nephrologist, dialysis nurse, dialysis technician, dietitian, and social worker. But the most important members of the health care team are the patient and the patients' family. By learning about the treatment, the patient can work with the health care team to get the best possible results, and lead a full, active life.

Here is what one nurse learned when she took on the challenge. Before starting up a PD program an application for a freestanding dialysis facility (form 855A) must be completed and forwarded to the Centers for Medicare and Medicaid Services (CMS). CMS approves the application and forwards it to the State of Michigan in Lansing for an official facility approval. The state department of surveyors evaluates the facility for the purpose of certification. Once the state finds that the facility is in compliance with the conditions of coverage for an End Stage Renal Dialysis (ESRD) facility, certification is granted and the facility is authorized to bill for services.[12]

After the facility is certified, a nurse, dietitian, social worker, and a receptionist must be hired. The medical space must be organized into a PD training room, a patient waiting area, a clean and soiled utility room, a break room, a laboratory area, a storage area, and a physician office.

Starting a dialysis center requires forming a partnership with a nephrologist, a physician specializing in kidneys and treating patients. In this case, Judy partnered with Dr. Boniface Tubie. Judith Adams, MN, FNP-C, and currently pursuing her DNP, had enough trust in herself and her physician to pursue her vision of starting a dialysis center and to trust that her actions and not her words would send the right message. As part of the learning process, she visited peritoneal centers to visualize operations and attended a weeklong course to learn how to train peritoneal patients.

Judith Adams: *In 2002, my supervising physician, Dr. Boniface Tubie, Nephrology and Internal Medicine, and I had a vision to start a peritoneal dialysis company, Great Lakes Dialysis LLC, in Detroit, Michigan. We both knew about peritoneal dialysis, but neither of us had experience starting up a dialysis program. We chose to establish a new program from scratch, learning and building the bridge as we walked on it. I was entrusted to initiate the program.*

I encountered many challenges as I contemplated deep change. The project exceeded all of my resources, but changing vision into reality is a test of one's vision, faith, and integrity. I began by learning all I could about peritoneal dialysis with the help of the Baxter trainers.[13] With their help, I was guided through state inspection and certification. I visited many peritoneal dialysis centers to visualize the operations and went through a weeklong course offered by the equipment company to learn how to train the peritoneal patients.

Finally the vision became a reality. After six months, the state inspection went off without a hitch, and we were open for business. The program grew by leaps and bounds, and within a year, we had fifteen functioning peritoneal patients. I hired a full-time peritoneal nurse, Anna Dimoglou, RN, who was entrusted to run the program. I kept the pride and momentum going by constantly engaging with Anna about what she could do to make her life and her patients' lives more rewarding. I conveyed to her that I cared about her and her contributions to the firm.

I then realized that we were spending far too much on supplies and looked to save money by changing product manufacturers. I switched product suppliers, procured the necessary training and resources to make the change happen, and saved a lot of money in the process.

We created a unity of purpose that pulled both of us forward with a shared sense of destiny, allowing us to achieve greatness and successfully build the program. Some patients drive over an hour to spend time with Judy and Dr. Boniface Tubie, they feel so strongly about their loving care that they are willing to bypass other dialysis centers just to go to Great Lakes Dialysis. The bridge was truly built as we walked on it.

Implementing Change in Fresh Ways

Montana Green, MS, RN, PCCN Associate Nurse Manager, Medical Progressive Care Unit, Beaumont Hospital, Royal Oak, helped nurses change the way they hand off vital information in front of both patients and their families. She learned that unless she changed the way she modeled her own behavior, she could not be effective in changing how her nurses behaved. She also visited other departments to see how they were responding to administration's mandated change in handoff procedures and how they supported their nurses and changed themselves.

Conveying information in front of the patient and his or her family during handoff improves patient safety and satisfaction. The impacts of less-than-ideal handoffs include delays in medical diagnosis and treatment, redundant communication, extra procedures and tests, lower patient satisfaction scores, higher costs, and less effective training for healthcare providers.[14] Patients transfer between diagnosis, treatment, and hospital care and may encounter three staff shifts each day, increasing safety risks at each interval. Communication about patients is vital, especially when transferring them from one type of care (outpatient, primary, emergency, surgical, rehabilitation, and hospital to home) to another.[15]

Incorporating situation, background, assessment, and recommendation (SBAR) can provide a standard communication framework for patient handovers. Encouraging the patient and his or her family to ask questions about the plan of care improves the effectiveness of handover communication. The patient and family remain the constant and can play a critical role in making sure continuity of care is practiced, particularly at hospital discharge. Collaborative (multidisciplinary) rounds are being used effectively to improve communication and ensure that patients and their healthcare provider are given key information regarding discharge diagnoses, treatment plans, medications, and test results. Here is how one nurse describes what she learned while working to role model open-communication behaviors with patients, families, and physicians.

Montana Green: *The offgoing and the oncoming nurses are expected to hand off vital information in the patient's room and in front of the patient and his or her family. Previously, nurses would exchange the information at the nursing station or in the unit's conference room. Nursing administration mandated that all units comply with this change. The goal of the change is to improve communication with patients regarding their plan of care, which is assessed by HCAHP* [Hospital Consumer Assessment of Health Plans] *survey sent to patients after their hospital stay.*

To date, the change has been only marginally successful. Reports are rarely given in front of the patient, and nurses often go outside the patient's room and exchange the report there. Nurses go into the patient's room to introduce the oncoming nurse and excuse the offgoing nurse. While there seems to be some positive feedback from patients about being able to identify their assigned nurse, there is no significant change regarding conveying the plan of care to patients and their families.

After reading about fear of change,[16] I talked to the nurses about what is expected, how they can make it work, and the possible benefits of integrating the change into their practice. One of my colleagues uses fear to force change: when she catches a nurse not complying, she reminds the staffer that she or he will be written up for not complying in the annual performance evaluation. However, I know that my colleagues and I have only changed our expectations and not our own behavior.

I know now that I need to change myself in order to change the circumstances on my unit. I plan to role-model the behavior of open communication with patients and families and step in to help out with patient care. I plan to reach out to other managers who have units that have successfully implemented this change and find out what made this change work for them and how they supported their nurses and changed themselves. I want to be open to thinking about this change differently and from other perspectives and to understand how to successfully implement bedside shift reports in a meaningful way. If I do not change, I cannot expect anyone else to change.

Accountable Care Organizations: Another Approach

The concept of accountable care organizations (ACOs) involves organizing and paying healthcare providers and suppliers in ways that encourage them to increase the efficiency, quality, and cost-consciousness with which they coordinate care. ACO providers then share in the savings this approach can produce.

The Nurse Practitioner Roundtable, which includes the American College of Nurse Practitioners (ACNP), the National Association of Pediatric Nurse Practitioners (NAPNP), the American Academy of NPs (AANP), the Gerontological Advanced Practice Nurses Association (GAPNA), and the National Association of Nurse Practitioners in Women's Health (NPWH), is a coalition of NP organizations formed to further the cause of all NPs by collaborating, unifying, and addressing issues of importance to NPs. The Roundtable submitted comments to the Centers for Medicare and Medicaid Services (CMS) on several major concerns regarding the ACO model:[17]

- *The ability of nurse practitioners to have their Medicaid patients aligned with an ACO, including ACOs established by NPs in autonomous practice*

- *Recognition of the qualifications of NPs to direct clinical management, quality assurance, and process improvements in ACOs*

- *Inclusion of NPs in internal processes for measuring clinical and service performance and use of the results to improve quality of care*

The Role of the APN in the Coming Decade

Elaine Webber is an assistant professor at the University of Detroit Mercy and former pediatric nurse practitioners at Botsford Hospital. While at Botsford, she started a pediatric lactation consultancy by working with patients and the pediatric physicians and eventually she was able to bill for her work. She pitched that Botsford offered better care because of this lactation service.

Elaine Webber: *I spent an afternoon this past week touring Michigan State University with my college-bound children.*

On the tour we were told that each "region" of student dormitories on campus had a health center for the student population along with one centralized Health Care Service for the entire student body. When the tour leader casually mentioned that all these health services were staffed by nurse practitioners, there wasn't a murmur or comment from the touring parents or students. It was a clear indication to me that the role of APNs appears to have become accepted as the norm—at least in the current generation of health care consumers. For me personally that was a thrilling moment. We have spent so many years fighting to get recognition for who we are, what we do, and what role we should play meeting the health care needs of a variety of populations. I finally feel that we have "arrived"—at least in the eyes of the public.

Looking toward the Future of Healthcare

Working together, physicians, NPs, and other healthcare providers can accomplish so much. Here are some examples of steps NPs have taken to effectively leverage their training and experience for the benefit of their patients, their employers, and their profession.

- Deanna Hays changed the way that nurse practitioners bill for their services. *"Insurance companies (particularly Medicare) require NPs to bill under their own provider numbers. Through many, many meetings with the legal department, physicians, and managers, we were able to get the NPs to start billing under their own provider numbers. NPs can now get credit for the primary care services they are providing."*

- Judith Adams stepped up to the plate and learned all she could about peritoneal dialysis, hired a consultant to help organize the plan, and adhered to all applicable policies and procedures in setting up the program. *"Finally the vision became a reality. After six months, the state inspection went off without a hitch, and we were open for business. The program grew by leaps and bounds, and within a year, we had fifteen functioning peritoneal patients. I hired a full-time peritoneal nurse, Anna Dimaglou, RN, who is now entrusted to run the program. She has done an exemplary job at growing and maintaining the program, and today, I only have to oversee it."*

- Montana Green changed her own behavior to role-model for her nurses how they could successfully implement bedside shift reports. *"I plan to role-model the behavior of open communication with patients and families and step in to help out with patient care. I plan to reach out to other managers who have units that have successfully implemented this change and find out what made this change work for them and how they supported their nurses and changed themselves. I want to be open to thinking about this change differently and from other perspectives and to understand how to successfully implement bedside shift reports in a meaningful way."*

- Elaine Webber felt pride in knowing that NPs run the clinics at Michigan State University and that after years of fighting to get recognition, NPs have arrived in the eyes of the public.

Together with physicians and other healthcare providers, NPs have an ongoing role to play in making meaningful changes in how healthcare services are provided and how treatment plans are rendered. Working in a team environment, such as the medical home model, allows NPs to see patients first and then refer those who need additional services to primary care physicians and then specialists. Transforming practices into a PCMH model requires a lot of work and dedication, but in the end it works. The PCMH model increases the incentives for cost control, but not at the expense of quality care.

Patient-centered care for all life stages and situations is based on a team approach. NPs function as a vital component of the healthcare world, providing services in multiple settings that include hospitals, acute care settings, primary care settings, rural health facilities, school health clinics, retail clinics, hospice and palliative care centers, cancer treatment centers, and operating rooms. NPs increase opportunities for expanding preventive care, to keep people healthy.

ACKNOWLEDGMENTS

This book belongs to the many, many people who thoughtfully helped me write its eight case studies. I wish to thank Dr. Joan Slager, Susan Imanse, Dr. Zylkia Rodrequez, and Mary Alice Martin from Bronson Women's Hospital in Kalamazoo, Michigan; the CEO and President of Hospice of Michigan in Detroit, Dottie Deremo, and Corporate Director of Innovative Programs, Roxanne Roth; Dr. Wendy Grube, Director, NP programs for the University of Pennsylvania in Philadelphia; Sandra Ryan, Chief Nurse Practitioner Officer, Take Care Health Systems (acquired by Walgreens in 2007), as well as Kathleen Gareth, Joyce Komori, Sue Ferbet, and Patricia Jacob. I am also indebted to Jonnie Hamilton, Director, Napoleon Jordan Center for HealthCare at Marcus Garvey Academy in Detroit, Michigan; and Dr. Laurie Hartman, Director of the Advanced Practice Nursing at the University of Michigan Hospital System and the School of Nursing in Ann Arbor, along with Melissa Baldwin, Erin Lindstrom, and Dr. Richard Prager. Further thanks go to Dr. Roz Harrison, St. John Macomb Hospital in Warren, Michigan, and Dr. Michael Dosch, Oakwood Hospital and Medical System in Dearborn, Michigan; and finally, to Dr. Lisa Chism, working for Karmanos Cancer Center in Detroit, Michigan.

I also wish to thank my family, including my son, Teren Lentz; daughter, Caryn Lentz; mother, Phyllis Solberg; and friend and partner, Boyd Chapin, Jr., for all of his time spent on this book. Last, I wish to thank my editor, Beverley DeWitt, who worked hard to provide me with her very best efforts.

CONTRIBUTORS

Dottie Deremo

As CEO and President, Dottie Deremo provides services to meet the emotional, spiritual, and physical needs of Hospice of Michigan patients and their families. Sydney's chapter on relationship building, end-of-care choices and expanding availability expands the thinking on what hospice means – living their last days, alert, pain free and surrounded by their loved ones.

Roxanne Roth

Roxanne Roth designs and develops the @HOMe Support™ Program, which was initiated under her guidance in the fall of 2006. Sydney's chapter teaches that all patients deserve the best care. Research both improves outcomes and reduces overall health care cost-savings by expanding services to one of our most vulnerable populations, those with serious and complex illnesses.

Wendy Grube

Dr. Wendy Grube teaches her students to treat rural women to listen to their concerns without judgment, and engage them in dialogues about their options for care. Sydney's chapter on empowering women with personal stories about their own experiences with breast or cervical cancer; these women deserve good cancer care with accurate, up-to-date information.

Sandra Ryan

Sandra Ryan is the chief nurse practitioner for Take Care Health Systems, a subsidiary of Walgreens. Sydney's chapter focuses on the expansion of the nurse practitioners into primary care, thereby promoting health and preventing disease. NPs and PAs working collaboratively with physicians provide coordinate, high-quality care at substantially reduced fees.

Jonnie Hamilton
Jonnie Hamilton is a nurse practitioner at Marcus Garvey Academy and a recognized expert in pediatric care. Sydney's chapter expands the focus to include clinical care, health promotion, disease prevention and health education, because of her there are fewer missed days of school, higher GPA scores, and she also counsels children and their families for asthma control.

Mike Dosch
Michael Dosch has worked at Oakwood Hospital and Medical Center in Dearborn Michigan since 2005. Sydney's chapter on the CRNA shows that caring for patient safely, discussing the plan of care, identifying good documentation, valuing timeouts, and identifying patient's identity, and building team cultures with nurses, surgeons and CRNA.

ABOUT THE AUTHOR

Dr. Sydney Lentz has extensive coaching and consulting experience in specialties including leadership assessment, senior team alignment, and managing change. She has coached numerous C-suite executives, including hospital CEOs, chief nursing officers, and physicians, as well as consulting with troubled hospital executive teams. She also serves as an adjunct faculty with Oakland University's Healthcare Executive MBA program and the School of Nursing, teaching courses on leadership and theory.

After receiving her PhD from the University of Michigan, Dr. Lentz began her career with General Motors in the organization development department in 1983. With more than 30 years in business, her background combines real-world executive experience with a strong track record of success that includes leading the coaching practice for a global HR consulting company and as a healthcare practice lead for another global organization.

Dr. Lentz's clients have included Karmanos Cancer Institute, Oakwood Health Care System, Henry Ford Macomb Hospital, Munson Medical Center, St. Mary's Healthcare, St. Joseph Mercy Oakland, Catholic Health Care Partners, The Mayo Clinic, Henry Ford Health System, Trinity Health System, physicians with the Health Alliance Plan, and the University of Michigan Surgery Leadership Development Program.

Dr. Lentz has published numerous articles on leadership and transforming healthcare and has spoken at national and international conferences on the topics of healthcare and healthcare leadership.

ENDNOTES

Chapter One

1. Hunnicutt, Susan. (2010). The U.S. Health Care System Needs to Change. Opposing Viewpoints: Universal Health Care. Detroit, MI: Greenhaven Press. Retrieved from http://find.galegroup.com/ovrc/printdoc. do?contentSet=GSRC&docT

2. Bohmer, Richard. (2010, April). Fixing health care on the front lines. Harvard Business Review, 88(4), 63-69.

3. Klein, Ezra. (2009). Do we have enough doctors for health care reform? The Washington Post. Retrieved from Voices. Washingtonpost.com/ezra-klein/2009/08/do-we-have-enough-doctors-for.html

4. Doty, M. et al. (2008, August). Seeing Red: The Growing Burden of Medical Bills and Debt Faced by U.S. Families. The Commonwealth Fund, Issue Brief. Retrieved from http://www.commonwealthfund.org/usr_doc/ Doty_seeingred_1164_ib.pdf?section=4039

5. Brandon, E. (2012). 65-and-older population soars: Florida and Arizona aren't the only places with large older populations. U.S. News and World Report. Retrieved from http://search.usnews.com/index_library/search?keywords=6 5+and+older+population+soars

6. Andrews, M. (2009, November 6). With doctors in short supply, responsibilities for nurses may expand. The New York Times, A18. Retrieved from http://prescriptionss.blogs.

nytimes.com/2009/11/06/with-doctors-in-short-supply-responsibilities-for-nurses-may-expand

7. Brook, R., & Young, R. (2010, April 21). The primary care physician and health care reform. JAMA, 303(15), 1535-1536.

8. Theiss, E. (2010). Will there be enough family care doctors to treat newly insured? The [Cleveland] Plain Dealer. Health Fact Check. Retrieved from http://blog.cleveland.com/metro/2010/04/will_there_be_enough_family_ca.html

9. How, S., et al. (2008). Public Views on U.S. Health System Organization: A Call for New Directions. The Commonwealth Fund, 11. Retrieved from http://www.commonwealthfund.org/Publications/Data-Briefs/2008/Aug/Public-Views-on-U-S--Health-System-Organization--A-Call-for-New-Directions.aspx

10. Reeves, L., et al. (2007). Substitution of doctors by nurses in primary care [Review]. Reprint of a Cochrane review, prepared and maintained by The Cochrane Collaboration and published in The Cochrane Library, 3, by John Wiley & Sons. Retrieved from www.cochrane.org/reviews/en/ab001271.html

11. Fairman, Julie, et al. (2011, January 20). Broadening the scope of nursing practice. New England Journal of Medicine, 364(3), 193-196. Retrieved from www.nejm.org/doi/pdf/10.1056/NEJMp1012121

12. The Cochrane Collaboration. (2008, August). SUPPORT summary of systematic review. Do nurse practitioners working in primary care provide equivalent care to doctors? Retrieved from www.who.int/rhl/effectivepractice_and_organizingcare/support_Task_Shifting.pdf

13. Associated Press. (2010). "Dr. Nurse? 28 States Seek to Extend Nurses' Power." Retrieved from http://www. aolhealth.com/2010/04/14

14. Naylor, Mary, and Kurtzman, Ellen. (2010). The role of nurse practitioners in reinventing primary care. Health Affairs, 29(5). Retrieved from http://web.pdx.edu/~nwallace/AHP/NPPC.pdf

15. Christensen, C., Bohmer, R., & Kenagy, J. (2000, September-October). Will disruptive innovations cure health care? Harvard Business Review OnPoint article. Purchased December 22, 2011, from www.hbr.org

16. Berwick, D.M., Nolan T.W., and & Whittington, J. (2008). "The Triple Aim: care, health and cost." Health Affairs, 27(3), 759-769. Summary of new health reform law. Retrieved from: http://content.healthaffairs.org/content/27/3/759.full.pdf+html

17. Newhouse, Robin, et al. (2011, September-October). Advanced practice nurse outcomes 1990–2008: A systematic review. CNE series. Nursing Economics, 29(5), 1-22. Retrieved from: https: www.nursing economics.net/co./2013/article300/02/.pdf

18. Institute of Medicine. (2010). The Future of Nursing: Leading Change and Advancing Health [Report brief]. Retrieved from http://www.iom.edu/Reports/2010/The-Future-of-Nursing-Leading-Change-Advancing-Health.aspx

19. Pohl, Joanne, et al. (2010, May). Unleashing nurse practitioners' potential to deliver primary care and lead teams. Health Affairs, 29(5). Retrieved from http://content.healthaffairs.org/content/29/5/900.full?ijkey=lXURzF1G6xJKw&keytype=ref&siteid=healthaff

20. Slager, Joan. (2004). Business Concepts for Health Care Providers: A Quick Reference for Midwives, NPs, PAs, CNSs, and Other Disruptive Innovators. Sudbury, MA: Jones and Bartlett Publishers.

21. Lugo, Nancy, et al. (2007, April). Ranking state NP regulation: Practice environment and consumer healthcare choice. The American Journal of Nurse Practitioners, 11(4), 8-24. Retrieved from http://www.eileenogrady.net/upload/Ranking%20of%20states%20AJNP_April_07_[final].pdf

22. Greene, J. (2012, February 17). Report: Overcoming primary care shortages essential to the future of health care. Crain's Detroit Business: Health Care Reform. Retrieved from http://miahec.wayne.edu/documents/dean-redman-on-primary-care-shortages-in-crains.pdf

23. Practicing Clinicians Exchange. (2012, March 21). Combined NP/PA workforce is 75% as large as the physician workforce. Retrieved from Newsbites@practicingclinicians.com

24. Help for Future Physician Assistants. (2012, March 25). NPs and PAs are reported to have 2 of the best jobs in America. Retrieved from http://pastudenthelp.blogspot.com/2012/03/nps-and-pas-are-reported-to-have-2-of.html

Chapter Two

1. Wikipedia. Retrieved from http://en.wikipedia.org/wiki/Nurse_midwife

2. Retrieved from http://www.bronsonhealth.com/FindADoctor/Practices/page964

3. Slager, J. (2004). Business Concepts for Healthcare Providers: A Quick Reference Guide for Midwives, NPs, PAs, CNSs,

and other Disruptive Innovators. Sudbury, MA: Jones and Bartlett.

4. King, T. (2006). Therapeutic moments. *Journal of Midwifery & Women's Health,* 51, 315-316. Article first published online 24 Dec. 2010. Retrieved from onlinelibrary.wiley.com.huaryu. kl.oakland.edu/doi/10

5. Welsh, J. (2011, July 10). C-section rates hit all-time high, study finds. Healthnews. msnbc.com. Retrieved from http://today.msnbc.msn.com/id/43807114/ns/today-today_ health/t/c-section-rates-hit-all-time-high-study-finds/#. T377wb9SRFA

6. Gegaris, C. (2007). Developing collaborative nurse/physician relationships. *Nurse Leader, (5)* 5, 43-46. Retrieved from http://www.sciencedirect.com.huaryu.kl.oakland.edu/ science/article/pii/S154146120700167X

7. Sullivan, M. (2010, July). Obstetric hospitalists could ease work burden. *Ob.Gyn News*, p. 2. Retrieved from http:// oblaborist.org/newarticles/2010_07_OBGynNews.pdf

Chapter Three

1. Brandon, E. (2012, January 9). 65-and-older population soars: Florida and Arizona aren't the only places with large older populations. *U.S. News and World Report*. Retrieved from http://money.usnews.com/money/retirement/ articles/2012/01/09/65-and-older-population-soars

2. Brawley, O. W., & Goldberg, P. (2011). *How We Do Harm: A Doctor Breaks Ranks about Being Sick in America.* New York, NY: St. Martin's Press. ISBN 978-0-67297-3. Kindle download.

3. The Business Journals. (2011, May 19). Hospice of Michigan program is "Just what the doctor ordered" to empower consumers. Detroit. PR Newswire. Retrieved from http://www.bizjournals.com/prnewswire/press_releases/2011/05/19/DC05072

4. Hospice of Michigan. (2012). Website: Home – Our Services. Retrieved from http://www.hom.org/?page_id=13

5. Hospice of Michigan. (2012). Website: Home – About Us – Vision, Mission and Values. Retrieved from http://www.hom.org/?page_id=129. Picture from the Hospice of Michigan Annual Report, Wednesday, February 6, 2011.

6. Goodman, D., et al. (2010). *Quality of End-of-Life Cancer Care for Medicare Beneficiaries.* Dartmouth Institute for Health Policy and Clinical Practice. Retrieved from http://www.dartmouthatlas.org/downloads/reports/Cancer_report_11_16_10.pdf

7. Kimbell, D., & Fowler, E. (2010, November 16). Nearly one third of Medicare patients with advanced cancer die in hospitals and ICUs; about half get hospice care. Dartmouth Institute for Health Policy and Clinical Practice. Retrieved from http://geiselmed.dartmouth.edu/news/2010/11/16_cancer.shtml

8. Astrow, A., & Popp, B. (2001, May 19). The Palliative Care Information Act in real life. *New England Journal of Medicine.* Retrieved from http://www.nejm.org/doi/full/10.1056/NEJMp1102392

9. Formiga, F., et al. (2004). End-of-life preferences in elderly patients admitted for heart failure. *QJM, 97*(12), 803. Retrieved from qjmed.oxfordjournals.org/content/97/12/803 and Fried, T.R., et al. (1999). Older persons' preferences for

site of terminal care. *Annals of Internal Medicine, 131*(2), 109-112. Retrieved from www.annals.org.huaryu.kl.oakland.edu/content/131/2/109.abstract

10. Kass-Bartelmes, B., & Hughes, R. (2003, March). Advance care planning: Preferences for care at end of life. *Research in Action,* Issue 12. Agency for Healthcare Research and Quality, U.S. Department of Health & Human Services. Retrieved from http://www.ahrq.gov/research/endliferia/endria.htm

11. Sach, G. (2000, November 15). Sometimes dying still stings. *JAMA, 284*(19), 2423. Retrieved from http://jama.ama-assn.org/content/284/19/2423.extract

12. Wikipedia. (2012). Caregiver. Retrieved from http://en.wikipedia.org/wiki/Caregiver

13. Felgen, J. (2004). A caring and healing environment. In M. Koloroutis (Ed.), *Relationship-Based Care: A Model for Transforming Practice* (Ch. 2). Minneapolis, MN: Creative Health Care Management.

14. Leininger, M. (2004). Five theoretical assumptions on caring. In M. Koloroutis (Ed.), *Relationship-Based Care: A Model for Transforming Practice* (Ch.1). Minneapolis, MN: Creative Health Care Management.

15. Van Hiel, A., & Vansteenkiste, M. (in press). Ambitions fulfilled? The effects of intrinsic and extrinsic goal attainment on older adults' ego integrity and death attitudes. *International Journal of Aging and Human Development.* Retrieved from http://www.selfdeterminationtheory.org/SDT/documents/2009_HielVansteenkiste_JAHD.pdf

16. McCarthy, E., et al. (2003, May 7). Hospice use among Medicare managed care and fee-for-service patients dying

with cancer. *JAMA, 289*(17), 2238-2245. Retrieved from: http://jama.ama-ssn.org/content/289/17/2238.full.pdf

17. Aspen Institute. (2012). Health span, not life span. Aspen Health Stewardship Project. Retrieved from http://www. aspeninstitute.org/policy-work/health-biomedical-science-society/health-stewardship-project/principles/health-span-not-

18. Quotes from Byock, I. (2004). *The Four Things That Matter Most: A Book about Living.* New York, NY: Free Press.

19. Thomas, A. (2009, April 9). WJR's Ann Thomas talks to Dottie Deremo, Hospice of Michigan CEO. Women Who Lead series [Audio podcast]. Retrieved from http://wjr.com/ Article.asp?id=1285542&spid=27945

20. Hospice of Michigan. (2012). Website: Home – About Us – What sets us apart. Retrieved 1 May 2012 from http://www. hom.org/?page_id=125

Chapter Four

1. West Virginia Breast and Cervical Cancer Screening Program. (2012, July 24). *Early Detection Is the Best Protection!* The impact of breast and cervical cancer. Retrieved from http:// www.wvdhhr.org/bccsp/detection.asp

2. Grube, W. (2008). *Science at Work in Rural Communities* [Unpublished document].

3. West Virginia Comprehensive Cancer Program. (2011, April 28). Mountains of Hope. Retrieved from http://www. wvcancer.com/AbouttheProgram/tabid/696/Default.aspx

4. West Virginia Breast and Cervical Cancer Screening Program. (2012, July 24). Retrieved from http://www.wvdhhr.org/bccsp/

5. Grube, W. (2012, August 3). Email. wgrube@nursing.penn.edu to sydney.lentz@gmail.com

6. Lengerich, E., et al. (2004, Spring). The Appalachia Cancer Network: Cancer control research among a rural, medically underserved population. Rural Health Research Models. *The Journal of Rural Health. 20*(2), 181-187. Retrieved from http://www.ncbi.nlm.nih.gov/pubmed/15085633

7. Walker, Jon. (2012, February 14). Level of Americans Without Health Insurance Continues to Rise. *MyFDL*. Retrieved from http://fdlaction.firedoglake.com/2012/02/14/level-of-americans-without-health-insurance-continues-to-rise/

8. Cornforth, T. (2009, November 8). LEEP Procedure. What is LEEP? – Loop Electrosurgical Excision Procedure. About.com. Retrieved from http://womenshealth.about.com/cs/surgery/a/leepprocedure.htm

9. Carone, D. (2001, October). A social cognitive perspective on religious beliefs: Their functions and impact on coping and psychotherapy. *Clinical Psychology Review, 21*(7), 989-1003. Retrieved from www.sciencedirect.com/science/article/pii/S0272735800000787

10. Grube, W. (2010, January 1). *Talk and Backtalk: Negotiating Cervical Cancer Screening among Appalachian Women in West Virginia.* Dissertations available from ProQuest. Paper AA134227. http://repository.upenn.edu/dissertations/AA13414227

11. Ward, A., et al. (2006, April). The impact of cancer coalitions on the dissemination of colorectal cancer materials to community organizations in rural Appalachia. *Preventing*

Chronic Disease, 3(2), 1-8. Retrieved from http://www.cdc.gov/pcd/issues/2006/apr/05_0087.htm

12. Centers for Disease Control and Prevention. (2002, June 21). Cancer death rates: Appalachia 1994–1998. *MMWR Weekly, 51*(24), 527-529. Retrieved from www.cdc.gov/mmwr/preview/mmrrhtml/mm5124a3.htm

13. Spencer, N. (2010, July). An epidemic of ill health among the poor: The social crisis in Appalachia. *World Socialist Web Site.* Retrieved from http://wsws.org/articles/2010/jul2010/app2-j24.shtml

14. Wikipedia. (2011). Bartholin's cyst. Retrieved from http://en.wikipedia.org/wiki/Bartholin's_cyst

15. Women in Government. (2010). New report on HPV and cervical cancer indicates states are turning challenges into opportunities for prevention efforts. Retrieved from http://www.womeningovernment.org/node/1038

16. Healthy women, informed. empowered. (2011). Retrieved from http://www.healthywomen.org/condition/human-papillomavirus-hpv?gclid=CKvd4vOd07ECFeEDQAodFEwAww

17. Papa, J. (2008). Effective healthcare communication. Retrieved from http://www.ehow.com/about_5421324_effective-healthcare-communication.html

18. Women in Government. (2010). New report on HPV and cervical cancer indicates states are turning challenges into opportunities for prevention efforts. Retrieved from http://www.womeningovernment.org/node/1038

19. U.S. Department of Health and Human Services, National Institutes of Health, National Cancer Institute. (2010,

November 22). *Mammograms* [FactSheet]. Retrieved from http://www.cancer.gov/cancertopics/factsheet/detection/fs5_28.pdf

Chapter Five

1. Cronenwett, L., & Dzau, V. (2010, April). *Co-Chairs Summary of the Conference, Who Will Provide Primary Care and How Will They Be Trained?* Josiah Macy Foundation. Retrieved from http://macyfoundation.org/docs/macy_pubs/JMF_PrimaryCare_Monograph.pdf

2. Theiss, E. (2010, April 5). Will there be enough family care doctors to treat newly insured? *The* [Cleveland] *Plain Dealer.* Health Care Fact Check. Retrieved from http://blog.cleveland.com/metro/2010/04/will_there_be_enough_family_ca.html

3. Brandon, E. (2012, January 9). 65-and-older population soars: Florida and Arizona aren't the only places with large older populations. *U.S. News and World Report.* Retrieved from http://money.usnews.com/money/retirement/articles/2012/01/09/65-and-older-population-soars

4. Pohl, J., Hanson, C., Newland, J., & Cronenwett, L. (2010, May). Unleashing nurse practitioners' potential to deliver primary care and lead teams. *Health Affairs*, 29(5), 900-905. Retrieved from http://content.healthaffairs.org/content/29/5/900.full.pdf+html

5. Retrieved from takecarehealth.com/Our_Care_Team.aspx

6. Rand Health. (2010). Health care on aisle 7: The growing phenomenon of retail clinics. Research Highlights. Retrieved from www.rand.org/pubs/research_briefs/2010/RAND_RB9491-1.pdf

7. Wikipedia. (2010). Convenient care clinic. Retrieved from http://en.wikipedia.org/wiki/ Convenient_care_clinic#cite_note-4

8. Mehrotra, A., et al. (2009, September). Comparing costs and quality of care at retail clinics with that of other medical settings for 3 common illnesses. *Annals of Internal Medicine, 151*(5), 321-329. Retrieved from http://www.rand.org/pubs/ external_publications/EP20090915.html

9. Weinick, R., Burns, R., & Mehrotra, A. (2010). Many emergency department visits could be managed at urgent care centers and retail clinics. *Health Affairs, 29*(9), 1630-1636. Retrieved from http://content.healthaffairs.org/ content/29/9/1630 abstract

10. Mehrotra, A., et al. (2008, September/October). Retail clinics, primary care physicians, and emergency departments: A comparison of patients' visits. *Health Affairs, 27*(5), 1272-1281. Retrieved from http://content.healthaffairs.org/ content/27/5/1272.full

11. Johnson, C. (2010, April 16). Facing doctor shortage, 28 states may expand nurses' role. The Associated Press. *USA Today.* Retrieved from http://www.usatoday.com/news/health/2010-04-16-nurse-doctors_N.htm

12. Fiercehealthcareeditors@fiercehealthcare.com. (2012). HHS supports community health centers with a $728M boost. Retrieved from https://mail.google/mail/ca/u/0#search/Fierc ehealthcare/1370ed4cb746dbc6

13. Convenient Care Association. (2010). *Convenient Care Clinics: High Quality Care* [Fact sheet]. Retrieved from www.ccaclinics.or/images/stories/downloads/factsheets/cca-factshet-quality-care.pdf

14. Patton, R., President, American Nurses Association. (2009, May 11). The role of primary care nurses [Letter to the editor, in answer to Pear, R., Shortage of doctors proves obstacle to Obama goals (2009, April 26)]. *The New York Times.* Retrieved from http://www.nytimes.com/2009/04/27/health/policy/27care.html

15. Newsbites@practicingclinicians.com. (2012, March 21). Combined NP/PA workforce is 75% as large as the physician workforce. Sources: U.S. Bureau of Labor Statistics. Career Guide to Industries, 2010-11 ed., Healthcare. Retrieved from http//www.bls.gov/oco/cg/cgs035.htm

16. Woodburn, J., et al. (2007, November/December). Quality of care in the retail health care setting using national clinical guidelines for acute pharyngitis. *American Journal of Medical Quality, 22*(6), 457-462. Retrieved from http://ajm.sagepub.com/content/22/6/457.abstract

17. Newhouse, R., et al. (2011, September-October). Advanced practice nurse outcomes, 1990-2008: A systematic review. CNE Series. *Nursing Economics, 29*(5), 1-22. Retrieved from https//www.nursing economics.net/ce/2013/article300/021.pdf

18. Reeves, L., et al. (2007). Substitution of doctors by nurses in primary care [Review]. The Cochrane Collaboration. Issue 3. Retrieved from: http://hss.state.ak.us/hspc/files/Primary_Care_Substitution.pdf

19. *EMR Return on Investment: Improving Efficiency and Quality with an Electronic Medical Record.* (2007). McKesson Empowering Healthcare. Retrieved from www.practicepartner.com/doc/EMR-Return-on-Investment.pdf

20. U.S. Department of Health and Human Services. (2012, May 1). Health care law helps community health centers build, renovate facilities, serve more patients [Press release]. Retrieved from http://www.hhs.gov/news/press/2012pres/05/20120501a.html

21. Aiken, L. (2011, January 20). Nurses for the future. *New England Journal of Medicine, 364*(3), 196. Retrieved from http://www.nejm.org/doi/pdf/10.1056/NEJMp1011639

Chapter Six

1. Rudavsky, S. (2010, May 30). School-based nurse practitioners help heal kids, keep them in class. *Indianapolis Star.* Indystar.com. Retrieved from www.Indy-star.com/article/20100530/NEWS1003/5300356/School-based-nurse-practitioners-help-heal-kids-keep-them-class

2. Weinick, R., Burns, R., & Mehrotra, A. (2010). Many emergency department visits could be managed at urgent care centers and retail clinics. *Health Affairs, 29*(9), 1630-1636.

3. Karp. H. (2009, June 10). Cracking the autism riddle: "Vaccine Theory" fades as a new idea emerges. Retrieved from http://www.huffingtonpost.com/harvey-karp/cracking-the-autism-riddl_b_219160.html

4. Willamina Elementary. (March 2011). School based health center, What's a nurse practitioner? Retrieved from http://sbhc.willaminak5.org/what-s-a-nurse-practitioner

5. Williams, G., et al. (2000). Extrinsic life goals and health-risk behaviors in adolescents. *Journal of Applied Social Psychology, 30*(8), 1755-1771. Retrieved from http://www.selfdeterminationtheory.org/SDT/documents/2000_WilliamsCoxHedbergDeci.pdf

6. Kasser, T., et al. (1995). The relations of maternal and social environments to late adolescents' materialistic and prosocial values. *Developmental Psychology, 31*(6), 907-914. Retrieved from http://www.selfdeterminationtheory.org/SDT/documents/1995_KasserRyanZaxSameroff.pdf

7. Wikipedia. (2012). Body mass index. Retrieved from http://en.wikipedia.org/wiki/Body_mass_index

8. Ryan, R., Patrick, H., Deci, E., & Williams, G. (2008). Facilitating health behavior change and its maintenance: Interventions based on self-determination theory. *European Health Psychologist, 10*(March). Retrieved from http://www.selfdeterminationtheory.org/SDT/documents/2008_RyanPatrickDeciWilliams_EHP.pdf

9. Lonsdale, C., et al. (2009). Self-determined motivation and students' physical activity during structured physical education lessons and free choice periods. *Preventive Medicine. 48*(1), 69-73. Retrieved from http://www.selfdeterminationtheory.org/SDT/documents/2009_Lonsdale_et_al_PreventiveMedicine.pdf

10. Teixeira, P., Patrick, H., & Mata, J. (2011). Why we eat what we eat: The role of autonomous motivation in eating behavior regulation. *Nutrition Bulletin, 36,* 102-107. Retrieved from http://www.selfdeterminationtheory.org/SDT/documents/2011_TeixeiraPatrickMata_NutrBul.pdf

11. Williams, G., et al. (2009). Reducing the health risks of diabetes: How self-determination theory may help improve medication adherence and quality of life. *Diabetes Educator, 35*(3), 484-492. Retrieved from http://www.selfdeterminationtheory.org/SDT/documents/2009_WilliamsEtAl_Diabetes.pdf

12. Wikipedia. (2012). Asthma. Retrieved from http:// en.wikipedia.org/wiki/Asthma

13. Brainy Quote. Dominique Wilkins. Retrieved from http:// www.brainyquote.com/quotes/quotes/d/dominiquew340878. html

14. Wikipedia (2012). Peak expiratory flow. Retrieved from http://en.wikipedia.or/wiki/Peak_expiratory?flow

15. Tree.com. (2011). Dust mites and asthma. Health & Wellness article. Retrieved from http://www.tree.com/health/asthma-safe-home-dust-mites.aspx

16. Wikipedia. (2012). Sickle cell anemia. Retrieved from http:// en.wikipedia.org/wiki/Sickle-cell_disease

17. Taras, H., & Potts-Datema, W. (2005). Obesity and student performance at school. *Journal of School Health, 75*(8), 291. Retrieved from http://faculty.ksu.edu.sa/almuzaini/ Important%20Resources/School-%20%D8%A7%D9%84% D9%85%D8%AF%D8%B1%D8%B3%D8%A9/school%20 performance.pdf

18. Centers for Disease Control and Prevention. (2010). *The Obesity Epidemic and United States Students: The 2009 National Risk Behavior Study.* Retrieved from http://www. cdc.gov/healthyyouth/yrbs/pdf/us_obesity_combo.pdf

19. School-Based Health Centers. U.S. (2010) U.S. Department of Health and Human Services. Retrieved from: http://www. hrsa.gov/ourstories/schoolhealthcenters/

Chapter Seven

1. Kleinpell, R. (2005, May). Acute care nurse practitioner practice: Results of a 5-year longitudinal study. *American Journal of Critical Care, 14*(3), 3211-3219. Retrieved from http://ajcc.aacnjournals.org/content/14/3/211.full

2. Leapfrog Group. (2012). Who we are. Retrieved from www.leapfroggroup.org

3. University of California San Francisco School of Nursing. (2012). MS Specialty Area: Acute Care Nurse Practitioner (ACNP). Retrieved from http://nursing.ucsf.edu/programs/specialties/acute-care-nurse-practitioner-acnp

4. Wikipedia. (2010). Teaching hospital. Retrieved from http://en.wikipedia.org/wiki/Teaching_hospital

5. University of Michigan School of Nursing. (2010, July 1). Dr. Hartman joins School of Nursing faculty. Retrieved from http://nursing.umich.edu/about-our-school/news-portal/201007/859

6. Fenske, C. (2011, October 20). *Leadership in Action* [Unpublished paper submitted to Nursing 820, Oakland University School of Nursing, to Dr. Sydney Lentz].

7. Scott, L., & Caress, A. (2005). Shared governance and shared leadership: Meeting the challenges of implementation. *Journal of Nursing Management, 13,* 4-12. Retrieved from http://scholar.google.com/scholar_url?hl=en&q=http://nursing.uchc.edu/shared_governance/docs/Shared%2520Governance%2520and%2520Shared%2520Leadership.pdf&sa=X&scisig=AAGBfm0C8j7YCiIl-0TGWh2gV0mUWh3PRQ&oi=scholarr

8. Lower, J. "Ski." (2011, October 27). *Engaging Your Staff: It Is More Than Just an Open Door Policy.* [PowerPoint

slides]. Paper presented at the annual Nursing Management Congress 2011, Las Vegas, Nevada. Retrieved from www. softconference.com/lww/sessionDetail/asp?SID=260057

9. Pfeffer, J. (2011, October 24). Don't dismiss office politics—Teach it. *The Wall Street Journal*. Retrieved from http://online.wsj.com/article/SB10001424053111904060604557

10. Rogers, C. (2005, June-August). Empathy. *Shift: At the Frontiers of Consciousness*. No. 7. Retrieved from http://media.noetic.org/uploads/files/S07_Empathy.pdf

11. Dunbar, B., Park, B., Berger-Wesley, M., & Cameron, T. (2007). Shared governance: Making the transition in practice and perception. *JONA, 37*(4), 177-183. Retrieved from http://www.ncbi.nlm.nih.gov/pubmed/17415104

12. Wikipedia. (2012). Attending physician. Retrieved from http://en.wikipedia.org/wiki/Attending_physician

13. Intensivist or hospitalist: What is the difference? (2010, January 15). Retrieved from thehappyhospitalist.blogspot.com/2010/01/intensivist-vs-hospitalist-what is.html

14. Reardon, K. (2005). *It's All Politics: Winning in a World Where Hard Work and Talent Aren't Enough*. New York, NY: Doubleday, Currency, 63.

15. Totterdell, P., et al. (1998). Evidence of mood linkage in work groups. *Journal of Personality and Social Psychology, 74*(6), 1504-1515. Retrieved from http://psycnet.apa.org/index.cfm?fa=buy.optionToBuy&id=1998-02892-007

16. Levinson, W., et al. (2006). How much do surgeons like their patients? *Patient Education and Counseling, 61*(3), 429-434. Retrieved from http://www.ncbi.nlm.nih.gov/pubmed/16024213

17. Tonges, M., & Ray, J. (2011, September). Translating caring theory into practice: The Carolina care model. *JONA, 41*(9), 374-381.

18. Dingman, S., et al. (1999, December). Implementing a caring model to improve patient satisfaction. *JONA, 29*(12), 30-37. Retrieved from http://journals. lww.com/jonajournal/Abstract/1999/12000/ Implementing_a_Caring_Model_to_Improve_Patient.7.aspx

19. Wikipedia. (2010). Grand rounds. Retrieved from http:// en.wikipedia.org/wiki/Grand_rounds

20. Wikipedia. (2010). Physician assistant. Retrieved from http:// en.wikipedia.org/wiki/Physician_assistant

21. Yarema, T., & Judy, J. (2011). Participation of an acute care nursing practitioner group in a medical-surgical intensive care unit: One hospital's perspective. *ICU Director, 2,* 25. Retrieved from http://icu.sagepub.com/content/2/1-2/25. abstract

22. Fry, M. (2011, March-April). Literature review of the impact of nurse practitioners in critical care services. *British Association of Critical Care Nurses, 16*(2), 58-66. Retrieved from www.ncbi.nih.gov/pubmed/21299758

Chapter Eight

1. Fosburgh, L., & Koch, E. (1995, April). The AANA Archives: Documenting a distinguished past [Imagining in Time column]. *Journal of the American Association of Nurse Anesthetists, 63*(2), 88-93. Retrieved from http://www.aana. com/newsandjournal/Documents/imagining_in_time_0495_ p088.pdf

2. American Association of Nurse Anesthetists (AANA). (2010, May). *History of nurse anesthesia practice.* Retrieved from http://www.aana.com/aboutus/documents/historynap.pdf

3. AANA. (2010, May). *CRNA profiles: Agatha Hodgins.* Retrieved from http://www.aana.com/resources2/archives-library/Pages/Agatha-Hodgins.aspx

4. AANA. (2011, June). *About us: Who we are.* Retrieved from http://www.aana.com/aboutus/Pages/default.aspx

5. McDowell, Marlene. (2010, Summer). *Nurse anesthesia: A specialty with endless opportunities.* Retrieved from http://www.minoritynurse.com/certified-registered-nurse-anesthetist-crna-anesthesia/nurse-anesthesia.

6. Fox, Kate. (2012, May 13). Ribbon cutting for former Cheboygan Memorial Hospital. Now called McLaren Northern Michigan, Cheboygan Campus. UpNorthLive.com. Retrieved from http://www.upnorthlive.com/news/story.aspx?id=753256#.UOcrdYnjlgk and http://www.mclaren.org/northernmichigan/CheboyganCampusnm.aspx

7. Monti-Seibert, E., Alexander, J., & Lupien, A. (2004, June). Rural nurse anesthesia practice: A pilot study. *AANA Journal, 72*(3), 181-190. Retrieved from http://www.aana.com/newsandjournal/Documents/181-190.pdf

8. Gunn, I. P. (2000, May). Rural health care and the nurse anesthetist. *CRNA, 11*(2), 77-86. Retrieved from http://www.ncbi.nlm.nih.gov/pubmed/11271044

9. Propofol (drug). (2009, August 7). *The New York Times.* Retrieved from http://topics.nytimes.com/topics/news/health/diseasesconditionsandhealthtopics/propofol/index.htm

10. Kelchner, Luanne. (2010). *Job duties for a CRNA.* eHow.com. Retrieved from http://www.ehow.com/list_6633990_job-duties-crna.html

11. Siemens USA. (2012). *Patient care documentation.* Retrieved from http://www.medical.siemens.com/webapp/wcs/stores/servlet/ProductDisplay?storeId=10001&langId=-1&catalogId=-1&productId=190964&catTree=,1008631,1025982,1025984, 1025967

12. Dunbar, Carol. (2004, August 9). *Top 10 tips for documenting patient care.* Nurse.com. Retrieved from http://news.nurse.com/apps/pbcs.dll/article?AID=2004408090315

13. Tenerife airport disaster. (2012). *Wikipedia.* Retrieved from http://en.wikipedia.org/wiki/Tenerife_airport_disaster

14. Joint Commission Center for Transforming Healthcare aims to reduce risk of wrong-site surgery. (2011, June 29). *Infection Control Today.* Retrieved from http://www.infectioncontroltoday.com/news/2011/06/joint-commission-center-for-transforming-healthcare-aims-to-reduce-risk-of-wrong-site-surgery.aspx

15. Rosenbach, M., et al. (1991, June). Study of nurse anesthesia manpower needs. *AANA Journal, 59*(3): 223-240. Retrieved from http://www.ncbi.nlm.nih.gov/pubmed/1950402

16. Hogan, P., et al. (2010, May-June). Cost effectiveness analysis of anesthesia providers. *Nursing Economics, 28*(3): 159-169. Retrieved from http://www.aana.com/resources2/research/Documents/nec_mj_10_hogan.pdf

17. Dulisse, B., & Cromwell, J. (2010, August). No harm found when nurse anesthetists work without supervision by physicians. *Health Affairs, 29*(8), 1469-1475. Retrieved from http://www.aana.com/advocacy/federalgovernmentaffairs/

Documents/No%20Harm%20Found%20When%20
Nurse%20Anesthetists%20Work%20Without%20
Supervision%20By%20Physicians.pdf

18. Gunn, I. (1996, December 1). *Journal of Clinical Anesthesia,*
    8(8): 683-685. Retrieved from http://www.deepdyve.com/
    lp/elsevier/the-proposal-to-certify-nurse-anesthetists-
    5slOnfh89O

19. Ray, T. (2007, October). Share your secrets—Teach! A
    proposal to increase the number of nurse anesthesia educators.
    AANA Journal, 75(5), 325-330. Retrieved from http://www.
    ncbi.nlm.nih.gov/pubmed/17966674

20. LocumTenens.com. (2011). CRNA salary. *2011 Compensation*
    and Employment Report. Retrieved from http://www.
    locumtenens.com/media/49325/2011-lt-crna-salary.pdf

21. Salary.com. (2012). *Salary Wizard:* Physician –
    Anesthesiology – U.S. national averages. Retrieved from
    http://www1.salary.com/anesthesiologist-Salary.html

22. Nurse anesthetist. (2011, March). *Wikipedia.*
    Retrieved from http://en.wikipedia.org/wiki/
    Certified_Registered_Nurse_Anesthetist

23. All-CRNA-Schools.com. (2011, June). *How to become a*
    certified registered nurse anesthetist (CRNA). Retrieved from
    http://www.all-crna-schools.com/certified-registered-nurse-
    anesthetist.html

24. Dunbar, C. (2004, August 9). *Top 10 tips for documenting*
    patient care. Nurse.com. Retrieved from http://news.nurse.
    com/apps/pbcs.dll/article?AID=2004408090315

25. Cowan, C., Vinayak, K., & Jasinski, D. M. (2002, June).
    CRNA-conducted research: Is it being done? *AANA Journal,*

70(3). 181-186. Retrieved from http://www.ncbi.nlm.nih.gov/pubmed/12078465

26. University of Detroit Mercy. (2013). About UDM. Meet our faculty. Mike Dosch. Retrieved from http://www.udmercy.edu/about/meet_faculty/chp/mike-dosch.htm

    A full list of schools offering CRNA programs can be found at http://www.aana.com/aanaaffiliates.accretation/Pages/Accredited.Programs.aspx

Chapter Nine

1. General Medicine PC. (2012, March). Welcome to General Medicine PC: An idea whose time has come! Medical directors, attending physicians and nurse practitioners for post-acute and long-term care. Retrieved from http://www.generalmedicine.com/

2. Lisa A. Chism, DNP, APRN, BC, NCMP, FAANP. (2012). Curriculum Vitae.

3. Karmanos Cancer Institute. (2011, March 22). Media Room. Karmanos breast cancer nurse honored as a fellow in nurse practitioner academy. Retrieved from http://www.karmanos.org/News/Karmanos-breast-cancer-nurse-honored

4. University of Tennessee Health Science Center. (2012). College of Nursing. Diane Todd Pace, PhD, FNP-BC, FAANP. Retrieved from http://www.uthsc.edu/nursing/faculty%20and%20staff/pace.php

5. U.S. National Library of Medicine. (2011, November 7). Vaginal dryness. Retrieved from http://www.ncbi.nlm.nih.gov/pubmedhealth/PMH0001894/

6. Karmanos Cancer Institute. (2011). Home/Patients & Visitors/Multidisciplinary Teams/Breast Cancer Program. Retrieved from http://www.karmanos.org/cancer-care/ teams/Breast-Team

7. Chism, L. A. (2013, February). *The Doctor of Nursing Practice: A Guidebook for Role Development and Professional Issues.* Burlington, MA: Jones & Bartlett Learning, ISBN 978-1-4496-4560-1.

8. Olsen, J., & Hanchett, E. (1997, Spring). Nurse-expressed empathy, patient outcomes, and the development of a middle-range theory. *Journal of Nursing Scholarship*, 29(1), 71-76.

9. Lisa-Kay Astalos Chism, DNP, APRN, BC, NCMP, FAANP. (2012, July). Curriculum Vitae.

10. Karmanos Cancer Institute. (2012, July 7). Media Room. Barbara Ann Karmanos Cancer Center opens Women's Wellness Clinic in Farmington Hills, Michigan. Retrieved from http://www.karmanos.org/News/ BarbaraAnnKarmanosCancerCenterOpensWomensWellness Clinic inFarmingtonHills

11. University of Michigan Health System. (2012). Sexual health. Retrieved from http://www.uofmhealth.org/medical-services/ sexual-health

12. American Association of Colleges of Nursing. (2011). Essential Series. Retrieved from http://www.aacn.nche.edu/ education-resources/essential-series

13. Ford, J. (2009, January 5). DNP coming into focus. *Advisor for NPs & PAs.* Retrieved from http://nurse-practitioners-and-physician-assistants.advanceweb.com/article/dnp-coming-into-focus.aspx

14. American Association of Colleges of Nursing. (2012, May). *DNP Fact Sheet*. Retrieved from http://www.aacn.nche.edu/media-relations/fact-sheets/dnp

15. Duke University School of Nursing. (2011). *Admission Requirements for Doctor of Nursing Practice (DNP) Program*. Retrieved from http://nursing.duke.edu/academics/programs/dnp/admission-requirements

16. University of Michigan–Flint. (2010). What sets UM-Flint's Doctor of Nursing Practice (DNP) program apart? Retrieved from http://www.umflint.edu/graduateprograms/programs/dnp.page

17. Online DNP Programs. (2010). Retrieved from http://www.onlinednpprograms.com/

18. Benner, P. (1984). From novice to expert: Excellence and power in clinical nursing practice. Menlo Park, CA: Addison-Wesley, pp. 13-34. Retrieved from http://www.health.nsw.gov.au/resources/nursing/projects/pdf/novice_to_expert_p_benner.pdf

19. Aiken, L. (2011, January). Nurses for the future. *The New England Journal of Medicine*, 364, 196-198. Retrieved from http://www.nejm.org/doi/full/10.1056/NEJMp1011639

20. Aiken, L., & Gwyther, M. (1995, May 17). The case for policy change. *JAMA: The Journal of the American Medical Association*, 273(19), 1528-1532. Retrieved from http://jama.jamanetwork.com/article.aspx?articleid=388479

21. Aiken, L., Cheung, R., & Olds, D. (2009, June 12). Education policy initiatives to address the nurse shortage in the United States. *Health Affairs*, 28(4), 646-656. Retrieved from http://www.ncbi.nlm.nih.gov/pmc/articles/PMC2718732/

For more information on advanced degree nursing education, also see:

allNursingSchools.com. (2013). Nurse Practitioner Programs and Career Resource Center: Your complete guide to nurse practitioner salary, careers, schools and degrees. Retrieved from http://www.allnursingschools.com/nursing-careers/nurse-practitioner/np

BestNursingDegree.com. (2013). Online Nurse Practitioner Programs. Retrieved from http://www.bestnursingdegree.com/programs/online-nurse-practitioner/

Chapter Ten

1. Benner, P. (2004, June). Using the Dreyfus model of skill development to describe and interpret skill acquisition and clinical judgment in nursing practice and education. *Bulletin of Science, Technology & Society*, 24(3), 188. Retrieved from http://bst.sagepub.com/content/24/3/188

2. Watson, J. (2009, Spring). Caring science and human caring theory: Transforming personal and professional practices of nursing and healthcare. *Journal of Health and Human Services*, 31(4), 466-482. Retrieved from http://www.ncbi.nlm.nih.gov/pubmed/19385422

3. Backer, L. A. (2007, September). The medical home: An idea whose time has come . . . again. *Family Practice Management*, American Academy of Family Physicians. Retrieved from http://www.aafp.org/fpm/2007/0900/p38.html

4. Forbes, J. (2012, August). 4 reasons why the medical home model will succeed. *The Care Transitions Journal*. Retrieved from http://www.finance.senate.gov/newsroom/chairman/release/?id=96d3e858-f5df-4764-b2b6-9ff18678e9ad

5. American Academy of Family Physicians. (2012). Primary care for the 21st century: Ensuring a quality physician-led team for every patient. Retrieved from www.aafp.org/online/en/home/membership/initiatives/nps/patientcare/pcmh.html

6. Starfield, B., Shi, L., & Macinko, J. (2005, October 3). Contribution of primary care to health systems and health. *The Milbank Quarterly*, 83(3), 457-502. Retrieved from http://www.commonwealthfund.org/usr_doc/starfield_milbank.pdf

7. United States Senate Committee on Finance. (2009, March 10). Health care reform from conception to final passage. Retrieved from http://www.finance.senate.gov/newsroom/chairman/release/?id=96d3e858-f5df-4764-b2b6-9ff18678e9ad

8. Nutting, P., et al. (2009, May). Initial lessons from the first national demonstration project on practice transformation to a patient-centered medical home. *American Family Medicine*, 7(3), 254-260. Retrieved from www.ncbi.nim.nih.gov/pmc/articles/PMC2682981/

9. Nurse Practitioner Roundtable. (2010, November). *Nurse Practitioner Perspective on Health Care Payment*. Washington, DC. Retrieved from http://www.nonpf.com/associations/10789/files/NP%20Roundtable-Reimb%20PolicyStatement2010.pdf

10. American Academy of Nurse Practitioners. (2012, September 19). AANP responds to the American Academy of Family Physicians report. Press Releases and Announcements. Retrieved from http://www.aanp.org/component/content/article/28-press-room/2012-press-releases/1082-aanp-responds-to-aafp-report

11. eHow. (2010). How to start a dialysis center. eHow.com. Retrieved from http://www.ehow.com/how_5050016_start-dialysis-clinic.html

12. Michigan.gov Home. Department of Licensing and Regulatory Affairs. End-stage renal disease facilities (ESRDs). Retrieved from: http://www.michigan.gov/lara/0,4601,7-154-35299_63294_27655_31217---,00.html

13. Baxter (2010). Peritoneal dialysis. Retrieved from: http://www.baxter.com/patients_and_caregivers/therapies/renal/home_dialysis/peritoneal_dialysis.html

14. Patterson, E., & Wears, R. (2010, February). Continuity of Care. Patient handoffs: Standardized and reliable measurement tools remain elusive. The Joint Commission. *Journal of Quality and Patient Safety*, 36(2), 52-61. Retrieved from http://www.handover.eu/upload/library/gv2g0z55seiol04iqcvai.pdf

15. The Joint Commission. World Health Organization. (2007, May). Communication during patient hand-overs. *Patient Safety Solutions*, 1(3), 1-4. Retrieved from http://www.ccforpatientsafety.org/common/pdfs/fpdf/presskit/PS-Solution3.pdf

16. Quinn, R. (1996). *Deep Change: Discovering the Leader Within*. San Francisco, CA: Jossey-Bass, a Wiley company.

17. National Organization of Nurse Practitioners Faculties. (2012, June). *Health Reform & Health Policy*. Retrieved from http://www.nonpf.com/displaycommon.cfm?an=1&subarticlenbr=25

INDEX